THE 3 WEEK PROGRAM
TO FEEL HEALTHIER, HAPPIER
AND BALANCED

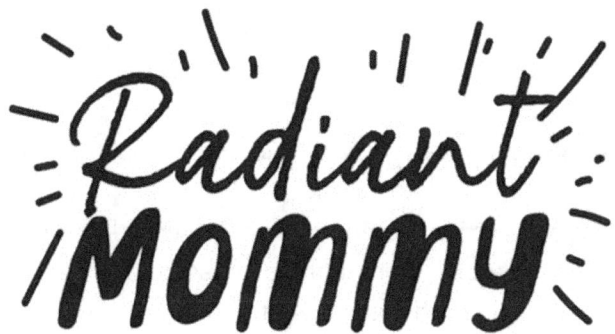

IXIANA HERNÁNDEZ WILMOT, MSHN

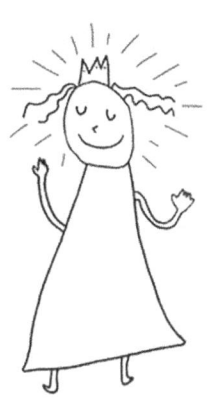

Copyright © 2020 by Ixiana H. Wilmot. All rights reserved.

This book or any portion thereof may not be reproduced or used in any manner whatsoever without the express written permission of the publisher, except for the use of brief quotations in a book review.

Strenuous attempts have been made to credit all copyrighted materials used in this book. All such materials and trademarks, which are referenced in this book, are the full property of their respective copyright owners. Every effort has been made to obtain copyright permission for material quoted in this book. Any omissions will be rectified in future editions.

Printed in the United States of America
First Printing, 2020

ISBN (Paperback): 978-1-7346800-0-3
ISBN (eBook): 978-1-7346800-1-0

Radiant Mami LLC
Clarksburg, MD 20871

www.radiantmami.com

CONTENTS

Dedication — 7
Disclaimer — 9
Introduction — 11

Part One: What Your Doctor Didn't Tell You About Stress — 15

CHAPTER ONE: Motherhood and Stress – Why Should You Care? — 17
- Enter the HPA Axis and the Stress Response — 18
- Tending to Your Garden — 21
- Diagnosing Stressors — 22

CHAPTER TWO: Stress, the Elephant in the Room — 25
- Perceived Stress — 26
- Circadian Disruption — 26
- Sugar Imbalances — 27
- Inflammatory Signals — 28

CHAPTER THREE: The Balancing Act — 31
- Creating Balance — 32
- Sleep — 32
- Detoxification — 33
- Nourishment — 37

Part Two: The Root of Health — 39

CHAPTER FOUR: The Power of Self-Love — 41
- So What Is Self-Love Exactly and What Does It Have to Do with Health? — 42

Connection to Self Leads to Self-Love 44
2-Minute Connection 45

CHAPTER FIVE: Training the Mind and
Creating Habits for Success 46
Tools for Creating a Positive Mindset 47

CHAPTER SIX: Accountability 51

Part Three: The Radiant Energy Program 53

CHAPTER SEVEN: Setting Up Goals 55

CHAPTER EIGHT: Week One: Restore Sleep 57
Step One: Set Up Your Bedroom 57
Step Two: Establish a Bedtime Routine 58
Step Three: Time Your Meals 61
Step Four: Balance Light Exposure 63
Step Five: Practice Gratitude 63

CHAPTER NINE: Week Two: Detoxification 65
Step One: Reduce Toxic Foods 66
Key Points About Sugar 70
Step Two: Reduce Your Toxic Load 71
Step Three: Be Mindful 73
Step Four: Hydrate 74
Step Five: Exercise 74

CHAPTER TEN: Week Three: Nourishment 78
Step One: Eat Colorfully 78
Step Two: Include Lots of Leafy Greens 79
Step Three: Supplement 79
Food Sources of Vitamin D 81
Step Four: Explore Food Sensitivities 82
Step Five: Do One Thing You Love That is Only for You .. 83

CHAPTER ELEVEN: Menu Planning — **85**
- Breakfast — 86
- Lunch — 88
- Dinner — 90
- Snacks — 92
- Transitional Foods — 93

Part Four: Feel Amazing and Live Amazingly — **95**

CHAPTER TWELVE: Radiant Mommy — **96**
- Connecting to the Goddess Within — 97
- The Investment and the Payoff — 98
- The Ripple Effect for You and Your Children — 99

Recipes — **101**

- Breakfast Recipes — 102
- Lunch Recipes — 107
- Dinner Recipes — 113
- Beverages and Broths for Radiant Skin — 122

About / Bio — **131**
Resources — **133**
Glossary of Terms — **137**
End Notes — **147**
Index — **155**

DEDICATION

To my grandmas, Ceci and Abuelita María, the strongest, fiercest women I know. To Terri, who has taken me as one of her own and lifts me up everyday with her kindness and support. But especially to my Madre Querida, my first love and the original Radiant Mami. Thank you for loving me so and teaching me to love myself.

DISCLAIMER

I am not a doctor. The information in this book is educational. It is not meant to diagnose, treat, prevent, or cure any disease and it is not a substitute for medical advice or treatment. Consult your physician if you suffer from any condition that requires you to follow a specialized diet or lifestyle protocol.

Note:

When working on some of the exercises in this book, keep in mind that you have access to downloadable worksheets and printouts through the Radiant Mami website.

If you would like to enhance your book experience with these free tools, use the link https://www.radiantmami.com/book-extras or select book extras from the book drop-down menu at www.radiantmami.com and enter the password: ICREATE

INTRODUCTION

Becoming a mother is an incredible thing, both beautiful and painful. It is the ultimate love affair sprinkled with unfathomable joy and a ton of WTFs?! Being a mom will have you feeling all the feels, all the time. It truly is a privilege and a superpower. For all the love and dedication you are going to put in for the rest of your days, you will have a legacy in this big world. You might have already heard that with great power comes great responsibility. If you are a mom, you know that is an understatement.

My favorite comedian, Jim Gaffigan, described parenthood by saying: "Imagine you're drowning and someone hands you a baby." This always resonated with me because all the hopes, dreams, and magic that come with motherhood are accompanied by an absurd amount of work. Sometimes it can feel like you are drowning. Sleepless nights, constant worrying, cooking, cleaning, organizing, negotiating, emotional availability, tech support, explaining, explaining again, finding items invisible to the naked eye, medical assistance, event coordinating, and overall supplier of all needs, are just a few of the jobs you will perform as a mother on a daily basis. It is stressful and can be lonely. You will be performing tasks to care for those around you every day and all that work will often go unnoticed. This invisible load of motherhood is often the cause of huge amounts of stress. And stress, particularly in huge amounts, will wreck your health.

When I became a mother, a part of me died. This sounds dramatic, but it is true. I slowly lost my sense of self, and that made it impossible for the new version of me that had been born with my child to grow. I was stuck and my health declined. One day, years later (I confess, it took me years to love my life as a mom), as I looked at my two children, something clicked. I do not know how to explain it, but I suddenly realized that the tired, cranky, sad, and uninspired version of me had to go. I wanted to be there with and for those kids I love so freaking much. I had to allow my new self to rise and I was determined to learn how. My life began to improve right then and there, and over the years I learned a lot about how to live my best life. With the support of my family, I went back to school to study nutrition and health. I became fascinated with how the body works. I especially loved learning about how hormones rule the body and how stress can throw a perfectly orchestrated hormonal system out of whack. It was incredible and empowering because within the process of learning I found myself again. I want to share this information with you because I want you to live your best life too. We do not need to do it the same way, but I hope the material in this book will help you find your own way. Maybe you got a little lost somewhere between that blissful moment you were handed your perfect baby and this morning when you ate a breakfast based on whatever your kids refused to eat. And as you look around exhausted and confused at the disaster zone that is your kitchen, you might be wondering: How did I get here?

You are not alone. Please know that you are not destined to a life without zest, energy, joy, and lovely skin. You are radiant and if you have lost some, or a lot, of that shine – chin up! – you can find yourself again in health.

Part of my journey led me to focus on stress and its repercussions on health. In my studies, I learned that the body regulates your response to stress via a system known as the hypothalamic-pituitary-adrenal axis or HPA axis. This system is involved in the fight or flight response, which helps your body act appropriately in case of an emergency. But the functions of the HPA axis are not limited to responding to stressors. The axis is also a part of energy production, temperature modulation, immune function, digestion, sexuality, and hormone balance. Mood, energy, libido, metabolism, immunity, cognitive function, and skin health are all affected by the HPA axis. If you feel like you need caffeine to get you through the day, if you feel uninspired, if you feel your skin has aged at the speed of light, and your kids are one "Mom!" away from becoming property of your in-laws, you could be suffering from poor HPA function.

HPA axis dysfunction is not talked about in Mommy and Me circles. It is not part of your yearly checkup protocol. And it is not the latest health news trend. I would like to help you get familiar with it because it is not uncommon and it could be affecting you.

This book will guide you on your journey to health. You will learn about the things that create stress in your body, how they affect your well-being and how to fix them in real and specific ways. I will explain the reasoning for each suggestion and give you the tools you need to take all the steps. The Radiant Energy program was designed by me based on my experiences with motherhood, what I learned from other moms, studies and my research. I wanted to create an accessible program that would help hardworking, busy moms take control of their wellness journey. I believe in you and your capability to transform your health, feel amazing and **love** your life. This program is a straightforward starting point to jumpstart your health makeover.

Motherhood will drive you to the edge of your seat, to the brink of madness and then, hopefully, back home to the love of your life and the greatest joy you have ever felt. You are entitled to your best life and I want it for you. Do you want it for yourself? This is it, ladies. The time has come to be your beautiful, vibrant self again. It will be my honor to get you started.

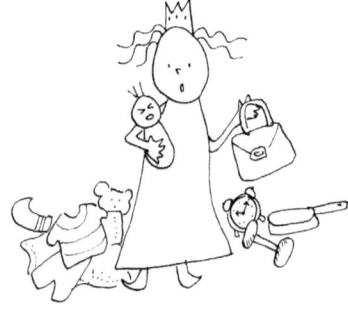

Part One

WHAT YOUR DOCTOR DIDN'T TELL YOU ABOUT STRESS

Stress promotes disease. It works relentlessly and vigorously, and you do not want to make enemies with it. Some forms of stress are necessary to sustain life; some are unavoidable. But if you allow stress to take the wheel, it will destroy your health. I cannot think of a single thing that is more damaging to your health than chronic stress. Chronic stress, the kind that lingers indefinitely, is at the root of disease. It creates inflammation, damages your cells, and breaks down entire systems, yet it often goes unattended. Why is that? How is it possible that stress, the cause of 90 percent of visits to primary care physicians,[1] is still an abstract concept to the general public?

The conventional approach to stress often relies on pills and ambiguous advice on how to manage stress. This path is unlikely to provide a clear picture of how stress affects you and what exactly you can do to address it. As a mother, you might have heard the very popular recommendation, "Get more rest" or its vague cousin, "Try to reduce stress." However well-intentioned, these suggestions are useless. How can we get more rest when we are so stressed out? How do we reduce stress when we don't even know the stressors that are affecting us? How do we deal with something we do not understand? This information is not discussed anywhere, and general practitioners have a tendency to dismiss women's symptoms of fatigue, poor mood or lack of vitality as an occurrence that comes hand-in-hand with motherhood. This lack of information and tools has left moms bound to suffer from the mysterious "motherhood disease" indefinitely. I would like to reassure you that fatigue, anxiety, moodiness, low libido, depression, inability to lose the baby weight, dull skin, and overall rapid aging are not normal components of motherhood. You are not meant to live like that.

Empowering women with the knowledge and tools to regain control of their health in a meaningful and sustainable way is long overdue. Your concerns about your health are not trivial. You are deserving of health. You are capable of understanding and managing stress. The first step is being informed. So let's begin, shall we?

Chapter One

MOTHERHOOD AND STRESS – WHY SHOULD YOU CARE?

Behind every super mom doing her best is a woman looking for balance. Unfortunately, creating and maintaining balance can feel like an impossible feat when you are up to your ears in mommying everything and everyone. A study published by *Sex Roles: A Journal of Research* demonstrated how the distribution of the mental and emotional work involved in managing the household and children, termed "invisible labor," affects women's health.[2] In the study, 90 percent of the women felt they carried almost all the responsibilities involved in the home, regardless of whether they had a partner that contributed to the household duties. Keeping track of the kids' extracurricular activities, stocking the pantry with snacks, making sure everyone has clean underwear and volunteering for school activities are all examples of invisible labor. In this study, most mothers felt solely responsible for their children's schedules and emotional health. Women reported feeling overwhelmed, having little time for themselves and feeling exhausted. Dear overworked mom, I see you, doing laundry while making dinner, composing a work email, and negotiating a peace treaty between your children.

Mothers are expected to excel in childcare, attend to the home and family, grow their career, keep social commitments, and maintain their physique. As you can imagine – or as you have probably experienced yourself – this impossible standards create a toxic amount of stress for mothers.

Perhaps you take pride in leading a stressful life and wear your hectic routine as a badge of honor. Perhaps it feels like this is what you are supposed to do as a mother or as a woman. And perhaps you have given up on living your best life in health because you believe being stressed, tired, and sick just comes with the territory. As a mother, a woman, and a wellness educator, I can tell you that is not the case. You are not supposed to feel stressed, tired, moody or unhealthy because you have joined the ranks of motherhood. Stress does not need to rule your life, emotionally or biologically.

Enter the HPA Axis and the Stress Response

In biological terms, stress is defined as a real or perceived disturbance of balance and the well-being of an organism. But stress can be necessary for survival. In a fire, for example, stress would activate the "fight or flight" response. This would provide you with the adrenaline and cortisol you would need to escape. After this, your body would return adrenaline and cortisol levels back to their natural state. The stress response would end there, allowing the body to resume normal functioning. But what would happen if, after you escaped the fire, another one started, and then, after reaching supposed safety, you found yourself face to face with a bear. Luckily, you probably won't find yourself in that situation any time soon. But if you did, your stress response would be in overdrive and eventually malfunction, throwing a wrench into other systems in your body. The system that handles the stress response is also involved in cardiovascular, metabolic, immune, behavior, and reproductive functions.[3] Repeat exposure to stressors is extremely detrimental to your health. This is not only true for fires or bear attacks, but also for what we are likely to encounter day-to-day.

Sugars, medication, over-exercising, lack of sleep, chemicals, pollution, toxic relationships, demanding jobs, and disease, like allergies, a cold or chronic conditions are all stressors. So, whether you stepped on a

Lego and injured your foot or you are having a never-ending argument with your toddler about why she shouldn't put her finger in the electric socket, your body will react to that event with a stress response, just like it would if you found yourself in a fire.

I want you to be familiar with stress, stressors and how the system works because information is power. Allow me to introduce you to a critical player when it comes to your health: The hypothalamic pituitary adrenal (HPA) axis. This system is driven by hormones that regulate the stress response. It consists of the hypothalamus, pituitary, and adrenal glands. The HPA axis is governed by the masterminds behind most body functions: hormones.

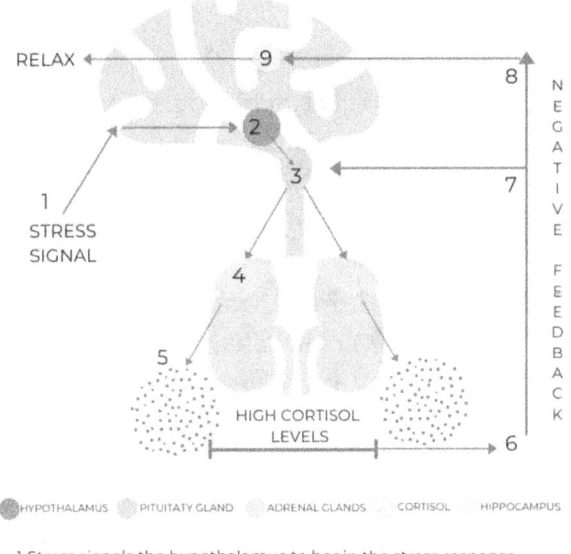

NORMAL HPA AXIS AND STRESS RESPONSE

● HYPOTHALAMUS ● PITUITATY GLAND ● ADRENAL GLANDS CORTISOL HIPPOCAMPUS

1. Stress signals the hypothalamus to begin the stress response.
2. The hypothalamus secretes CRH to stimulate the pituitary.
3. The pituitary gland secretes ACTH to stimulate the adrenal glands.
4. Stimulated by ACTH the adrenals release the stress hormone cortisol into the bloodstream.
5. High levels of cortisol in the bloodstream deal with the stressor and cause a negative feedback.
6. The negative feedback signals the brain to conclude the stress response, as the stressor has been dealt with.
7. High cortisol levels signal the pituitary gland to stop production of ACTH, so cortisol release can be suspended.
8. High cortisol levels also signal the hippocampus to inform the brain that the stress has passed, and it is time to restore the body to its natural calm state.

When confronted by a stressor, your brain reacts by releasing corticotropin-release hormone (CRH) in the hypothalamus. CRH stimulates the pituitary gland to produce adrenocorticotropic hormone (ACTH). ACTH signals the adrenals to make and release the stress hormones cortisol and DHEA. These hormones go all around your body signaling various mechanisms, such as increasing sugar levels so your body can produce lots of energy to run or attack. Once the stressor has passed, the system goes back to baseline by what is called negative feedback. Negative feedback occurs when high cortisol levels in the blood signal the hypothalamic-pituitary unit to decrease levels of CRH and ACTH. This causes cortisol levels to drop back to normal. You are safe, the stress was dealt with, and your body goes back to its business of digesting food, defending against a virus, or whatever was happening before the stressor crashed the party.

When you are under chronic stress (lots of fires and bear attacks, real or imaginary), cortisol levels remain high for a prolonged period of time. This can desensitize cortisol receptors in the body. As a result, the negative feedback becomes dysfunctional, because it does not react even to high levels of cortisol. So your body is constantly in a state of panic, which affects all body functions. The cells, organs, and pathways involved in the stress response are the same ones that keep you healthy through digestion, detoxification, fertility, the immune system, the menstrual cycle and the hormonal system. If the body is put in a position to choose what to attend to first, it will *always* choose stress, therefore neglecting everything else. This is why imbalances in the HPA axis, such as those brought on by chronic stress, can produce symptoms commonly associated with aging,[4] along with inability to lose weight, anxiety, fatigue, irritability, depression, and unhealthy skin.

So what does this all mean? Well, ignoring symptoms like fatigue, moodiness, unhealthy skin, weight gain, insomnia, and impaired cognitive function can really mess up the HPA axis. This means that your hormones will suffer greatly and because your hormones are catalysts to almost all body functions, so will your health.

Tending to Your Garden

Women are amazing. They are capable of creating human beings, birthing them, feeding them, tending to all their material and emotional needs while often being part of the workforce, and taking care of a home. Almost 70 percent of American mothers hold a paid job outside of the home.[5] Unfortunately, working moms have little societal support in the United States. A study by sociologist Caitlyn Collins found the U.S. to have the worst support for working mothers. In her research, she found that American mothers were more prone to experience crushing guilt and work-family conflict.[6] Without societal and sometimes partner support, mothers adjust by changing jobs, sacrificing sleep and personal time, and putting their health at the bottom of their to-do list. A survey of 3,000 American women reinforces this point as it found that 72 percent would always put their needs last and that 1 in 4 was dissatisfied with their overall health.[7] This is an alarming number, and you should take note because you might be one of them.

For all the work they do and the pivotal role they play in society, there is little effort put into keeping mothers healthy. This isolation can make them feel lost, anxious, and dissatisfied with their lives. Guilt and the pressure to be the perfect mother affect women's health regardless of whether or not they subscribe to intensive motherhood ideals.[8]

Imagine that you have a beautiful garden. Now imagine that you started planting weeds in that garden every day. What would your garden look like by the end of a month or a year? This is what happens to your body when you allow stress to take over. Excessive stress equals an inflamed body which creates more stress, brewing a perfect storm for accelerated aging and disease. At this point, I would like to ask you to take a minute to examine your garden. Is your garden being taken over by weeds? If this is the case, if you feel like your beautiful, healthy self is being covered by a layer of dullness and tension, it is time to start weeding the stress out.

Let's start working on that right now. In order to address stress, it is important that we are able to identify it. Use the following exercise to identify some of the stressors in your life.

Diagnosing Stressors

On a scale from 1 to 10, 10 being the highest, rank the following stressors:

1. **Family:** caring for your child, relationship status, family demands, taking care of the home, etc.

2. **Work/Finances:** job satisfaction, co-workers, boss, demands and expectations, career growth, financial responsibilities and compensation.

3. **Social:** interactions, engagements, expectations and roles within your community.

4. **Emotional:** personal traits, fears, anxieties, personal expectations, traumas, rumination, etc.

5. **Health:** disease, weight concerns, low self-esteem, rapid aging, lack of energy, allergies, etc.

6. **Environmental:** pollution, excessive noise, lack of space, exposure to chemicals, unpleasant surroundings, extreme temperatures.

Use the chart below to help you spot the areas that might be causing the most stress in your life.

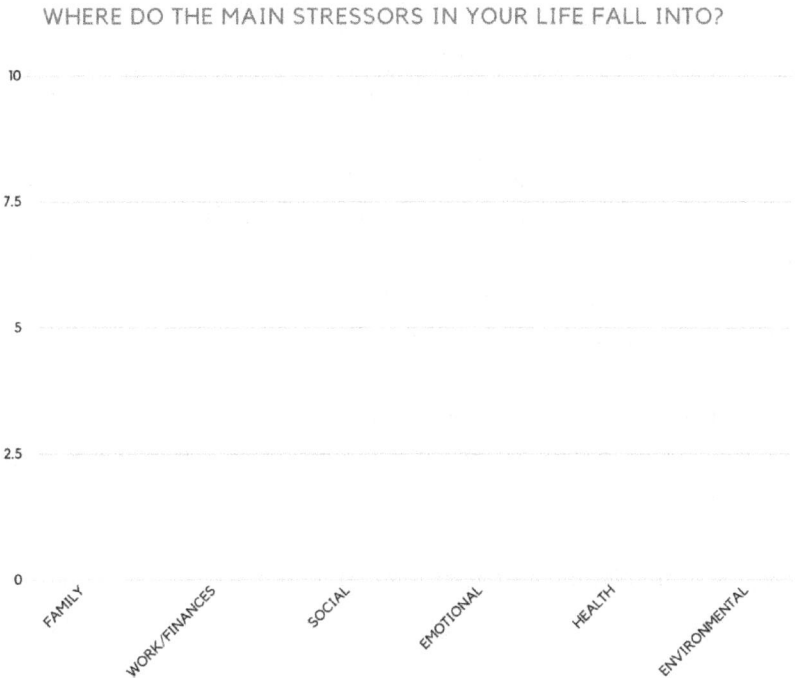

Once you have identified the highest ranking stressors, I would like you to make a list of the things that cause you stress under those categories. For example, if family is one of the top stressors, list the specific trigger points, like worrying about your child's reading skills. Your list could look something like this:

Family
- partner won't help with house chores
- arguing with my 10 year old about homework

Work
- boss is unreasonable
- I do not earn what I deserve

Emotional
- I am constantly using negative self-talk

Environmental
- one hour drive to work

Once you have a list, it will be easier to visualize things that might otherwise go unnoticed and unattended. You will also see that some of these stressors can be eliminated. Let's say your partner's lack of participation in household chores drives you nuts. In order to address this, you can make time to have a calm conversation with them about why their help would mean so much to you and find some chores that they would be willing to help with on a regular basis. This would alleviate some of your load and take away that stress from your daily routine.

Some stressors can't be eliminated completely but maybe they can be reduced. If you have to drive one hour to work every morning, you can start listening to an audio book to make your commute more pleasant. The point of this exercise is to bring daily stressors into the light. This will help you find solutions to manage the amount of stress these situations bring into your daily life.

Chapter Two

STRESS, THE ELEPHANT IN THE ROOM

According to the American Institute of Stress, 77 percent of people regularly experience physical symptoms caused by stress. The American Psychological Association found that 49 percent of women surveyed in America reported that their stress levels increased in a five-year period. The most reported sources of stress include money, work, family responsibilities, and health.[9] Mothers are especially susceptible to chronic stress given the high demands involved in raising a family.

Everyday activities including feeding, bathing, and transporting children can cause fatigue, frustration, and confusion, even when parenting children who are calm and even-tempered.[10]

Linking back to the HPA axis and how its dysfunction affects your overall health, there is a solution. It can actually be corrected in most cases by modifying stress signals coming from perceived stress, circadian disruption (problems with sleep-wake cycles), sugar imbalances, and inflammation.[11] So you *can* manage stress and improve your health. You can regain balance. You can tame the stress elephant; I know you see it. You can protect your HPA axis, thus restoring your vitality, by addressing stress signals. With this in mind, let's explore some high-profile stressors individually.

Perceived Stress

Perceived stressors are those that are set off by non-physical stimuli from outside the body, like a traffic jam, a crying baby, or your child's inability to pee inside the bowl. This type of stress has more to do with your perception of the event, not with how harmful or dangerous the event is. A recent study shows that underlying a mother's burnout symptoms was a craving for perfection, a lot of self-pressure, and a tendency to anticipate their children's future needs. Their stressor was mostly fear that ranged from not being a good enough mother to losing control and their sense of self. Participants reported that due to perceived stress and anxiety, they would experience intense fatigue.[12] These types of stressors activate hormonal pathways that result in several behavioral and physiological responses like anxiety, low libido, depression, and inflammation.[13]

Techniques like cultivating gratitude, which I will provide instructions on in the next chapter, have shown to lower depression and perceived stress.[14] Psychological interventions and distractions that improve expectations before stress have been shown to influence the response to perceived and biological stress, and reduce the cortisol response after an acute stressor.[15] That means that your mindset has a direct correlation to how your body reacts to stress at a very real and biological level.

Circadian Disruption

The circadian rhythm refers to all the physical, mental and behavioral changes that take place during the 24-hour daily cycle. According to research, long-term circadian disruptions are linked to chronic conditions such as premature mortality, obesity, impaired glucose tolerance, diabetes, psychiatric disorders, anxiety, depression, and cancer progression.[16] Short-term disruptions are associated with fatigue, reduced cognitive function, and overall impaired wellness.[17] In mammals, circadian rhythms are generated and synchronized by a central clock in the hypothalamus.[18] This clock adapts to signals called zeitgebers.[19]

Light and dark cycles are the most important zeitgebers. When our eyes receive light, our bodies sync into solar time. The light and dark cycles of the day and night regulate your circadian rhythm. Scheduled exposure to light and darkness are critical to keeping your circadian rhythm in balance. Proper exposure to light, especially in the mornings, can help reset the internal clock. This is why it is so important to make sure you get enough sunlight during the day and reduce exposure to light, including artificial lighting, at nighttime.

Meal timing is another zeitgeber. Timed meals perform an important role in synchronizing circadian rhythms.[20] Consuming meals at consistent times every day helps regulate your internal clock. Consuming meals late in the evening should be avoided as it adversely impacts sleeping, insulin sensitivity and metabolism.[21] This is very important because in combination with the HPA axis, the circadian rhythm causes cortisol fluctuations throughout the day that influence sleep-wake cycles, hormonal regulation, eating patterns, digestion, body temperature, and metabolism. These varying hormone patterns are responsible for maintaining a healthy stress response, energy production, and mental clarity.[22] In order to re-establish and support the circadian cycle, timed or scheduled exposure to light and darkness and regularly timed meals are critical.

Sugar Imbalances

Stress and HPA axis dysfunction are considered high-risk factors in obesity-driven chronic disease.[23] A stressful situation leads to the release of cortisol via the adrenal glands. Cortisol is designed to increase energy in the short-term in order to deal with stressors; it does this by blocking insulin secretion. This helps maintain a high level of glucose (sugar) circulating in the blood which is used for energy. When stress presents itself, glucose is needed to produce lots of energy quickly so we can fight or take flight. Insulin is a hormone secreted by the pancreas and its main job is to manage sugar levels in the blood. In the presence of cortisol, insulin production is put on hold so that glucose can be readily available. When stress is prolonged, insulin function is affected. In the long run, this constant interference between cortisol and insulin could lead to insulin resistance, inhibition of insulin secretion and disruption of normal functions of insulin in the body.[24]

Problems with insulin function are a big component of metabolic syndrome. Metabolic syndrome is a condition that encompasses several disorders that increase your chances of chronic diseases like diabetes and heart disease. There is significant evidence suggesting progressive dysfunction of the HPA axis with elevated levels of circulating cortisol is related to excess fat in the abdomen and type 2 diabetes.[25] Obesity and metabolic disorders have a complicated cause-and-effect relationship with stress disorders.[26] So stress can cause obesity, metabolic syndrome, diabetes, and heart disease, and these diseases further stress your body.

A diet high in sugars combined with a sedentary and high-stress lifestyle is a terrible combination as it disturbs your body's normal functioning and causes disease. Research shows that visceral adiposity (excess fat in the abdominal area) and insulin resistance (when your body cannot properly utilize insulin) can be resolved in part by balancing the stress response.[27] This fact suggests that issues with insulin (like obesity, type 2 diabetes, brain fog, anxiety, and fatigue) could be corrected by reducing stress and supporting the HPA axis.

Inflammatory Signals

Inflammation always gets a bad rap, but it is an important tool in immune function and one of the mechanisms your body uses to protect you against infections or injuries. If you broke a bone, inflammation would prevent you from moving that area as you normally would, giving your body time to heal. Just like the stress response, it is a component of health as long as it is balanced. But when inflammation becomes a regular occurrence, illness ensues. Low-grade chronic inflammation is extremely problematic and is promoted by repeated stressors.

Inflammation in the body is controlled by hormones like cortisol and adrenaline. They either increase or inhibit pro-inflammatory signals.[28] Adrenaline increases inflammation, while cortisol reduces inflammation.

When the body is in a state of chronic stress, chronic inflammation occurs. This state of excessive inflammation creates a continuous activation of the HPA axis increasing cortisol activity; over time, this suppresses immune functions,[29] hence the link between stress and disease via malfunction of the immune system.

Inflammation can be considered a stressor because if it is persistent, it will subdue HPA axis function. This creates complications with cortisol production and sensitivity. Without proper cortisol function, inflammation cannot be controlled. Your body will be in a state of constant inflammation, which will make you sick.

Many conditions can cause chronic inflammation. Food allergies, intestinal permeability, imbalances with your gut bacteria, autoimmune conditions, asthma, and metabolic disorder can all lead to chronic inflammation if they are not addressed. Excessive inflammatory response causes an increased production of some very destructive molecules called free radicals.[30] Free radicals are unstable molecules that damage other molecules in the body and create oxidative stress (OS).[31] OS is associated with rapid aging due to the accumulation of damage to lipids (fats), proteins and DNA.[32] These components of inflammation are like drunk rock stars trashing a hotel room, and the hotel is your body. They will age your skin, reduce your energy, adversely affect your mood, increase irritability, and promote poor memory and cognitive function – not to mention they will make you sick. Chronic inflammation and its components can also cause the classic symptoms of the elusive "motherhood disease": fatigue, poor mood, low libido, and dull skin.

Antioxidants, often found in fruits and vegetables, help neutralize free radicals. This is one of the reasons a diet high in fruits and vegetables is so important. Supporting detoxification and antioxidant production in order to avoid excessive buildup of free radicals will facilitate healthy inflammatory function.

Correcting HPA axis dysfunction by reducing and addressing stressors via diet and lifestyle modifications is an important step in ensuring health. If you want to feel and look your best, you cannot ignore the damaging effects of stress in your life. It is time to switch roles, from passive observer to active participant, and take charge of your health.

Chapter Three

THE BALANCING ACT

So far you have learned about the ways stress affects your body and how it impacts your health. Now you will learn how to address stress and create balance in your body.

Creating balance is the main goal in wellness. The natural state of our minds and bodies is balance. The mind and body cannot thrive in discord. We are all unique and need different things to be happy and healthy. Balance is the one constant.

It is important to understand that balance does not mean that nothing ever moves or changes. Movement, adjustments, and change are part of creating balance. Imagine yourself standing in the ocean and feeling your body shift as the waves hit you. You are still standing but you are constantly adjusting. Sometimes the waves will be bigger and rougher; this is part of the experience of being in the ocean. But even then it is possible for you to remain standing *and* enjoy the ocean. Allowing movement while focusing on your center, being mindful, and paying attention to your body's cues will keep you from being dragged by the waves. Balance is something we must practice and work with constantly. It requires commitment, but it is worth it because balance will always bring you back to health. Balance will grant you *your* best life, whatever that is.

Creating Balance

The body is a wonderfully smart creation. Every single hormone, cell, organ, and system has a purpose. Every part of your body is designed to work in synergy. In this harmonious state, your health blooms.

As you have learned, the stress response – and its right hand, the HPA axis – is crucial in keeping your body in balance. So what can you do to achieve balance? Well, luckily your body already has a PhD on how to function optimally. It just needs you to take purposeful action.

As a woman and mother of two, I know how precious your time is. The multitude of things we need to juggle is quite astounding, and for that please make sure you pat yourself on the back on a daily basis. For the sake of making your transformation into your best self a realistic and sustainable endeavor, we will focus on three pillars of health you can work with. Sleep, detoxification, and nourishment are the backbone of this program and your allies in your journey to health.

Sleep

Sleep is fundamental to health. Unfortunately, chances are you are not getting enough. A study published by the American Academy of Neurology estimates that less than half of mothers get enough sleep regularly and most are tired throughout the day.[33] According to the National Sleep Foundation (NSF), the average woman aged 30 to 60 only sleeps 6 hours and 41 minutes a night. If you are a mom, you are probably sleeping less. The NSF says you should be getting between seven and nine hours a night.[34] While it is normal to be sleep-deprived during the beginning of motherhood, prolonging this pattern of poor sleep for years will sabotage your health.

Regular sleep disturbances negatively affect circadian rhythm by disrupting normal function of your body's biological clocks. These clocks can be found in nearly every organ and are controlled by a master clock in the brain. The master clock can be severely impacted by irregular sleep-wake patterns, throwing off your body's 24 hour cycle. This creates imbalance because your circadian rhythm regulates most biological and behavioral functions in your body. Simply put, without proper sleep, health is not possible. Supporting the circadian rhythm promotes hormonal balance in the HPA axis, allowing the body to regulate itself and get restful sleep. Going to bed at a consistent time and waking at the same time every morning is one of the easiest ways to support circadian rhythm. Nutrients like magnesium, potassium, tryptophan, omega 3s, antioxidants, and b-vitamins promote relaxation and the health of the nervous system. In Chapter Eight, I will provide a detailed guide to improve your sleep.

Detoxification

Substances that cause bodily harm are considered toxic, and they are not limited to chemical elements. They also encompass environmental factors like overly critical co-workers, negative TV programming, and draining relationships. Because of the burden they pose to the body, consider them stressors. Susceptibility to toxic substances is influenced by the body's chemical load and the function of the detoxification system, among other factors like age and disease.[35] Problems in the detoxification system affect hormones, immunity, the nervous system, and metabolism. This creates imbalances that lead to inflammation, a stressor I mentioned earlier. Inflammatory signals activate the HPA axis and lead to more stress and toxicity in the body.

In order for inflammation to subside, the triggers must be removed. This includes foods, household cleaners, personal hygiene and beauty products, toxic relationships, and negative environmental factors.

Let's say you step on a nail. How would you treat this? Would you put a bandage over the nail and take some aspirin? Of course not; you would remove the nail and then do the bandage and aspirin. You would remove the nail because it is the only way your foot would be able to heal. If you left the nail in your foot, it wouldn't matter how many bandages, ointments, and pain killers you used, that injury would never heal. Not only would it not heal, but would become infected and it would spread. Eating a diet high in toxic foods, using harmful chemical-laden products, entangling yourself in destructive relationships, and allowing tons of negativity in your life while trying to support detoxification is like trying to heal your foot without removing the nail.

Nutrient-Depleting Substances

The first step when using nutritional support to promote detoxification is removing foods and beverages that contribute to the total body burden of toxins.[36] Added sugars, damaged or trans fats (those that have been heat processed and are usually found in fried foods), and refined foods containing additives, preservatives, and colorings should be removed or significantly reduced. These substances are nutrient-depleting because they can interfere with nutrient absorption, create toxicity, and use up the nutrient storages in your body.

According to the U. S. Department of Agriculture, 57 percent of the American diet comes from processed foods, and only 11 percent comes from whole foods.[37] Making a shift from a diet based in refined foods to a clean diet can be challenging, and it takes time. Your objective should be to introduce healthier eating habits and remove the junk in the process. Adding more fruits, vegetables, and whole foods rich in fiber promotes healthier eating habits because they make you feel satisfied and nurtured. This makes the process of eliminating nutrient-depleting foods, like sugar, easier. Eliminating added sugars (those that do not occur naturally in foods) alone is a huge game changer when it comes to nurturing your body. It is a catalyst for profound change. In Chapter Nine, I will explain in more detail how sugars affect your health.

While you are adjusting to changes in your diet, you can use transition foods. Transition foods are those that contain less junk than their counterpart. For example, you could replace regular potato chips with organic potato chips cooked in coconut oil. These types of foods can be used as a safer alternative to foods that are very high in damaging components like added sugars, unhealthy fats, and artificial colors and flavors. Any step you can take toward reducing depleting foods is valuable. Ultimately, eliminating these food offenders will have the most impact.

In order to support detoxification, reduce inflammation, and maintain balance, an anti-inflammatory diet is recommended. A diet based on whole grains, fruits, vegetables, healthy fats, adequate protein, and natural spices supports detoxification. Foods high in antioxidants, phytonutrients (health-promoting natural chemicals found in plants), minerals, and fiber should be favored. Whole foods like broccoli, cabbage, kale, berries, garlic, and spices like turmeric have a supportive effect on body detoxification.[38] These can help regulate the inflammatory process; with less inflammation, there is less toxicity in the body and vice versa. Grocery lists and menu plans are provided in Part 3 of this book. The importance of adequate water intake will also be discussed. Clean drinking water is a must for health. It is necessary for flushing toxins, maintaining electrical balance within body ions, and for cell nourishment and repair.[39] Beverages like coffee, sweetened drinks, soda, and alcohol dehydrate the body and contribute to toxicity. They should be consumed sparingly.

Environmental Toxins

Toxins in the environment are also worth noting. Let's focus on household, beauty, and personal hygiene products. One of the most significant avoidable toxic burdens for women is beauty products. According to a national survey, the average American woman uses 16 beauty products a day![40] Beauty products can contain reproductive and developmental toxins such as phthalates and heavy metals, yet the information available to the public is often limited and inconsistent.[41] The skin absorbs these toxic chemicals, and they go directly into the blood, acting as hormone disruptors. Learning about what chemicals to avoid when purchasing products you use at home and on your body is important. Finding sources for safer alternatives is a life saver. I will show you how to do this in Chapter Nine.

The Toxic Mind

Toxicity is not only found in the things we put on and in our bodies. It also comes from the thoughts we allow in our mind and the information we interact with. This is not an esoteric concept. As you have learned, the stress response is activated whether the stressor is physical or perceived. Your reaction to any situation will have a deeper impact on your HPA axis than the situation itself.[42] Constant negative thinking or rumination supplies stress mechanisms with a lot of fuel.[43] This affects you by coloring your perception of everyday events. Daily stressors become more difficult for you to deal with. As a result, your body's ability to remain in balance is jeopardized. Repetitive negative thoughts and interactions result in overstimulation of the HPA axis, causing the nervous, endocrine and immune systems to malfunction.[44]

A negative mindset is toxic and makes it very difficult for you to feel happy, establish healthy patterns and support health. Multiple studies suggest that mindset is a distinct and meaningful variable in determining the stress response. Mindset determines whether stress is enhancing or debilitating.[45] Developing a positive mindset is as vital as proper water intake when it comes to creating lasting wellness. You cannot live a positive healthy life if you sustain a toxic, negative mindset.

The silver lining is that there is an abundance of ways you can create a positive attitude. Meditation, mindfulness, gratitude, exercise, breathing purposefully, and focusing on the good are just a few examples. In Part 2, I will guide you through the process of optimizing your mindset for success and health.

Nourishment

Nutrition is fundamental for health. It will come as no surprise to you at this point that it is all about balance. Nutrients work synergistically. A variety of nutrients are required to promote health. Minerals like calcium, magnesium, sodium, potassium, and zinc are involved in HPA axis function and moderate metabolic effects of stress.[46] Studies show that omega-3 fatty acids support the immune-inflammatory system, the HPA axis, and the autonomic nervous system.[47] Maintaining a supply of these nutrients is fundamental to regaining health, the balance of the HPA axis, and overall well-being. Bone and vegetable broths, avocados, coconuts, dark leafy greens, and nuts are a few examples of foods to include. Reducing the glycemic impact (the effect of sugar in the blood) on the diet will also aid in maintaining hormonal balance. Eating breakfast within two hours of waking, having regular meals, and avoiding added sugars and highly processed foods are all important components of a healthy HPA axis.

Vitamins, minerals, fats, carbohydrates, protein, antioxidants, and water all play a fundamental role in sustaining optimal wellness. A diet that includes all of them supports balance. Foods that deplete the body of health, like added sugars, damaged fats, and synthetic substances, should be replaced with nutrient-dense alternatives.

I will not be taking you down the calorie rabbit hole in this book. When you eat a diet rich in whole, nutrient-dense foods and you practice mindfulness, you do not need a calorie calculator. The main purpose of this book is to help you reduce stress so you can create balance and live your best life. Balance requires love, dedication, and quality nutrition, not counting calories.

Nurturing, a fundamental aspect of nourishment, is all about connection, self-love, and self-respect. Health-powered foods are a reaffirmation of our commitment to ourselves and a way of expressing self-love. But health is not only related to the foods we eat. As we discussed earlier, health has everything to do with the way we treat ourselves, the company we keep, the relationships we nurture, and the thoughts we allow in our minds. Creating distance from toxic relationships and behaviors is a part of nurturing. Making time to do the things that bring joy, health, and love into our lives is at the beginning and the end of any successful wellness effort. Are you ready to put yourself at the top of your to-do list and make the adjustments that will bring you incredible change? I encourage you to take the leap. Your amazing life is waiting.

Part Two

THE ROOT OF HEALTH

Motherhood can be isolating. After I had my first child, I found myself experiencing a kind of loneliness I had never known before. There I was with my beautiful healthy baby, a loving partner, a supportive family, and the financial means to stay at home. Yet I fell into depression, completely lost my sense of self, and became an extension of my child. The person I had grown to know over the years was disappearing, and I felt an emptiness that made sense to no one. I slowly abandoned myself and assumed it was just what happens when you become a mother. This led me to a number of health problems over the following years. I was a functioning adult but I felt lost, tired, unmotivated, and struggled to stay afloat. My body and mind were aging rapidly on account of the incredible stress I was experiencing and the lack of self-care. Three years later I had a second child. I took forever to conceive because of my health mishaps, and I wondered if this was it for me. A life surrounded by love and beauty that I couldn't truly enjoy. What was missing? Granted, I was exhausted by the demands of a newborn, but it was more than that. It was not just lack of sleep. The biggest pitfall, I came to realize eventually, was that I had disconnected from myself. I was a kite without a string. I was at the mercy of every situation because I had no anchor. Because of that, everything was a thousand times harder to accomplish. I had disconnected from my body, and my body got sick.

When we get overwhelmed with responsibilities, we start placing ourselves at the bottom of our to-do list in order to make space for everything else. We minimize our needs, we ignore our body, and we neglect our spirit. We might not realize it immediately, but over time every ounce of your being will beg you to re-connect by presenting you with discomfort, dissatisfaction and disease.

Connection is your biggest advocate for wellness. It is the kite string. In connection you are present and aware. It is through connectedness that you can truly see what is in front of you. It grants you the capacity to witness where you are without harsh judgement. Connection allows you to accept what is happening and know what needs to change. When you are connected, you are seen, in your entirety, with the flaws that make you so precious and all your spectacular beauty. With connection comes balance, and with balance comes health.

It is in your own light that you will find health, joy, love, and wealth. Believe it; you are just what you need.

Chapter Four
THE POWER OF SELF-LOVE

The concept of self-love is not something we learn about at school. For many it is not taught at home either. Throughout our lives, we long for love without realizing we can provide it to ourselves.

My mother tried her best to teach me about self-love. She told me every day how wonderful, perfect, and deserving of love I was. To this day, I am not sure why I struggled for decades to understand that my worth was not in the eyes of others but my own. I ached to feel loved unconditionally by others and always fell short of their expectations, no matter what I did. This warped sense of self drove me to countless relationships that broke my heart. But most devastating was the effect it had on my opinion of the world, myself and my health. It was not until my late 30s that I really understood the power of self-love. It took a severe depression, exacerbated by the demands of motherhood, and a number of health issues to understand I needed to find and love myself as hard as I loved my children. I was tired all the time. I was sad, anxious and angry. I yelled at my children and lashed out at my partner. My skin was unhealthy and itched constantly. My immune system was weak, and I was completely lost. I had no motivation or drive. I felt helpless and alone; even though I was surrounded by love, I just didn't know how to love myself. I saw doctors who dismissed my suffering and assured me it was just exhaustion and stress, which they attributed to motherhood. Aside from routine tests and a prescription for vitamin D, I was left to just deal with it because that is what mothers do.

But I started to question, is it? Is that what mothers do? Are mothers supposed to ignore symptoms that indicate hormonal imbalances, nutrient deficiencies, and an overactive nervous system? Was I supposed to adapt to survival mode? Was I supposed to accept I had lost my vitality, health, and joy? No way! I did not know all the answers – I still don't – but that seed of self-love that my mother planted in me when I was a child bloomed, and it saved my life. It was self-love that led me to take charge of my well-being. It took time, trials and errors, and a lot of compassion and adjusting, but I turned my life around. Now I can tell you with confidence that I know you are capable of incredible things, like transforming your life.

The answer to your optimal, best, healthiest life is YOU. I want you to repeat this to yourself and engrave it in your mind; you are what you need. You can change your life to whatever you want your life to be. It takes work, commitment, tools, knowledge, and support, but most importantly it takes a lot of self-love. And this is a lesson you do not want your child to miss out on. All the abundance, love, health, and joy you want for your child, you must want for yourself too. If you feel they deserve all the beauty this life has to offer, know that you deserve it too. If you love yourself that hard, your child will learn that they can do the same.

So What Is Self-Love Exactly and What Does It Have to Do with Health?

I believe self-love is the ability to bestow on yourself the kind of respect, kindness, and care you would wish for those you love unconditionally. Being a mother gives you the opportunity to become a nurturing expert. Tending to all the needs of a tiny human will provide you with wisdom and an amazing capability to love selflessly. It will also grant you sleep deprivation, tons of responsibilities, and stress. Yes, stress and discomfort are part of motherhood, but they do not define it. You define it, and the way you see and treat yourself will write that definition for you. The amount of self-love – or lack of it – will set the stage and it will either prevent or promote health.

Your habits are a reflection of the way you feel about yourself. So take notice, because what you see might surprise you and not always in a good way. Creating healthful habits can be challenging, mostly because we have a tendency to put ourselves last. As mothers, we are taught that our children and our family come first. As lovely as this concept might sound, I think it is overrated and ultimately wrong. I am not bashing the importance of family or the privilege it is to care for your child. Your children and your family are important, but they are not more important than you. Think of it this way: If you have no interest in caring for yourself, what will your children learn from that? If you are constantly neglecting your wants and needs, what message does that send to your child? Not only that, but if you fail to attend to yourself, you will inevitably lose your health, physically and emotionally. How can you give your family the best if you are a hot mess? You can't.

Self-love is not just bubble baths and retail therapy. Self-love is making yourself a priority so you can honor your body by incorporating habits that enhance your health. Think of the ways you try to encourage your child to practice a skill or create a habit you know is crucial for their well-being. Let's use oral hygiene as an example. You ask your child to brush their teeth every night. You explain that it is important for healthy teeth and avoiding painful cavities. Your child might complain about it, but every night you remind them of why it is so important. Every night you try to show them how to do it correctly. You do this, despite their protests, because you know this is a habit that will support their well-being. Not learning this important skill will negatively impact their lives. You make them brush their teeth because you love them. My question to you is, do you brush your teeth every night? Are you willing to practice the skills that will support your well-being? It can be difficult to get past the discomfort that accompanies adjustment and change. But just like brushing your teeth every night, it is an act that with practice and commitment will become a healthful habit. Self-love is about seeing the opportunity to grow and heal and taking it, even if it takes some practice.

Self-love will push you to stick to habits, and those habits are what will allow you to experience your best life. You are meant to live an amazing life, and it begins with the love you grant yourself.

Connection to Self Leads to Self-Love

When you connect with yourself, you will have your best interest at heart because you understand your worth. When you connect with yourself, you will find it easy to connect with others without losing yourself. You will understand the universe is here for you, and you are part of it all. You will live with purpose, and you will be able to ground yourself.

Begin by connecting with you, and obstacles will become treasured lessons. With connection, establishing habits that create and sustain health will be a joyful endeavor.

Connect and listen. Your body will tell you all you need to know. That is how powerful you are.

If this all seems foreign to you, you will need to work on it. Just like you work on bonding with family and friends, your connection will deepen with the time and love you put in. There are many ways to help you connect with yourself. Meditation, breathing exercises, noticing your surroundings and reactions, or simply observing yourself in silence are a few ways you can start bonding with yourself. You can also try this brief exercise and modify it according to your wants and needs.

2-Minute Connection

Close your eyes and place your hands on your heart.

Feel your heart beating. How does it feel?

Now notice your breath. Is it fast and shallow? Is it slow and deep? How does it feel?

With your hands still on your heart, take a deep breath. Inhale for four seconds.

Notice how the air fills your lungs.

Exhale slowly to the count of eight.

Notice how the air leaves your lungs.

Repeat this a couple of times.

Then allow your breath to return to autopilot.

Keep your eyes closed for another minute and notice how your body is taking care of you. Your heart is pumping, your lungs are purifying, blood is transporting, and all your systems are doing their best to keep you safe.

How do you feel? Do you feel grateful? Do you feel trust? Do you feel love? Do you feel admiration? Do you feel change? What do you feel?

Listen to your answer.

Open your eyes and say "thank you" for the lesson.

Chapter Five

TRAINING THE MIND AND CREATING HABITS FOR SUCCESS

All your experiences and actions are influenced by your mindset; your mindset rules your world because it connects you to you. Researchers suspect that positive thinkers are better protected against the inflammatory damage of stress.[48] Studies also find that negative emotions are associated with a weaker immune response.[49] Have you ever experienced an upset stomach when under stress or a "gut" feeling when under pressure? This is because your gut is covered by a network of neurons creating the enteric nervous system, also known as the second brain. The enteric nervous system and the central nervous system communicate bi-directionally,[50] controlling fluid secretion, blood flow, muscle activity, and other functions. When the stress response is activated, the functions of the enteric nervous system are put on pause. This can lead to abdominal pain and discomfort. If the stress response is persistent, the digestive system is disrupted, and gastrointestinal disorders may occur.[51]

Rumination (chronic attention to affliction, its causes and its consequences) is associated with behaviors that focus on negativity. Negative thoughts can be perceived as stress. According to research, when rumination is inhibited, perceived stress decreases.[52] If we rewire our thought process to focus on positive feelings routinely, instead of negative ones, our amount of perceived stress will lessen significantly. Imagine that! Such a simple concept could have a massive impact on your health.

Tools for Creating a Positive Mindset

Allowing negativity to control us is a form of self-sabotage. Do not fall into this trap. If you have persistent negative thoughts, become a detective. Explore the reasons behind these feelings; find the root, observe it, and forgive it. Let go of that heavy burden and move forward with gratitude for the lessons learned. Shifting our consciousness and focus to the gifts in our lives can help diminish negative stressors and create balance. A transformation in consciousness to focusing on the blessings rather than misfortunes can balance the negative thoughts that stem from personal stressors.[53] Gratitude, mindfulness, kindness, and affirmations are tools you can use to take control over negativity and transform it into healthful habits.

Gratitude

Clinical trials indicate that gratitude has a powerful impact on health. Gratitude impacts your emotional health, reducing the risk of anxiety, substance abuse, and depression. It also supports your HPA axis by promoting immune function and normal blood pressure.[54] In order to reframe your mind, you must adopt an attitude of gratitude.

A simple exercise to cultivate this is a gratitude journal. Keep a small notebook by your nightstand and every evening before you go to sleep, write three to five things you are grateful for that happened that day or in general. Other examples of making gratitude a part of your daily routine are:

- **Expressing one thing you are grateful for during dinner time.** Everyone at the table says one thing they are grateful for that day. It is a beautiful way to bond with your children and teach them about gratitude.

- **Say "thank you"** before you put your feet on the ground every morning, and make sure to say it out loud. This simple exercise will help get your day started in a positive way. I also recommend that you make it a habit to say thank you to yourself while looking in the mirror; be grateful to yourself. Practice using the words to thank others for the things they do, big and small. Be grateful for nature, your home, the grocery store, books, pets, food, and events. Everything, even the hard times, serves a purpose.

Mindfulness

The concept of mindfulness has been defined in many different ways. In the context of this book, mindfulness refers to being present in a state of non-judgmental awareness. Mindfulness is connection with the self. As a therapeutic technique, mindfulness can be used to silence judgement and allow you to experience a situation without an emotional attachment to the outcome or situation itself. Mindfulness is meant to reduce suffering, promote positive feelings, and enhance your life experience.[55]

Meditation is the preferred method for pursuing mindful awareness. But this might not be something that comes easily to you. You might feel like you do not have time to meditate; you might see it as a foreign concept; you might think it is boring or you simply have no idea how to do it. Fortunately, there are numerous resources that make meditation a simple exercise you can fit into your schedule. Apps, articles, videos, and audio files are readily available at the click of a button. A meditation as short as two minutes, like the one on page 45, in the morning could have a powerful impact on your day. I understand how hectic and busy life can get; but if you are not willing to open yourself to a different perspective, if you cannot make time to care for yourself, the transformation you long for will not happen. Meditation has been studied for its beneficial effects on pain, blood pressure, irritable bowel syndrome, anxiety, depression, and insomnia, amongst other conditions.[56] It is a very influential habit.

Kindness

Current research shows a link between kindness and altruistic behaviors with health and longevity.[57] This is chemical, via hormones and neurotransmitters, and centered around oxytocin. Often termed "the love hormone," oxytocin has an impact on behaviors, including promoting feelings of well-being and mitigating the stress response.[58]

As chronic stress impacts health by accelerating the rate of cellular aging,[59] it could be said that cultivating kindness contributes to longevity by preventing the acceleration of aging at the cellular level.

Affirmations

Science has found that our brains can be rewired through our thoughts. Your thought patterns affect your brain activity, which in turn affects your actions. The purpose of creating positive affirmations is to reprogram your mind and create a positive mindset that will help you reach your goals. There is a large body of evidence demonstrating that self-affirmations can reduce stress, increase well-being, and make people more open to behavioral change. Research shows that neural activity brought on by self-affirmations can have an impact on the choices we make toward our health.[60]

Negative thoughts have the power to control situations, especially if they are repetitive. Harboring negativity is a sure way to sabotage your chances of success. Negative thoughts become self-fulfilling prophecies, which are extremely destructive to health. In order to give yourself a boost of inspiration, I want you to write your own affirmations and use them daily. Here is a simple guide.

Creating Your Affirmations

When you write your affirmations:

1. Use the words "I" or "I am".
2. Write in the affirmative. For example: "I am making the right choices now." vs. "I am not going to make mistakes."
3. Write in the present tense: " I am doing this with ease."

Sample Affirmations

- I am full of positive thoughts from the moment I wake up.
- I enjoy thinking positively, and it feels natural.
- I am creating my best life.
- I support my body by listening to it and giving it what it needs to thrive.

Using the information above, create your own affirmation or set of affirmations. Create them in an empowered tone, even if you do not feel so empowered right now. Remember this exercise is meant to help you reframe your thoughts and train your brain. Use a pen and paper to write them. Once you have created your affirmations, repeat them to yourself every morning. Whenever you feel a negative thought is starting to take over (it is okay to have negative thoughts as long as you are able to observe them and then release them), repeat your affirmations. Write your affirmations five times on a piece of paper or in your gratitude journal; do this as often as you can. Use your phone and record your affirmations, then play them to yourself before bed or at any time you feel you need to hear them.

Through repetitive thinking, writing, listening and reciting, your positive affirmations will train your brain and give you the best chance at success.

Chapter Six

ACCOUNTABILITY

You are in charge of your life. Not me, not your children, not your family or friends. You are the only one who can determine if you are going to reach your goals or not. This book is meant to guide you and inspire you. I know you are capable of change. I know you can feel amazing and live your best life. I believe that with fierce conviction, but I cannot do it for you nor can anybody else. At this moment, I want you to acknowledge the power within you. Know that you are a force of action and creation. You can tap into that force, always, because it is within you and for you.

Accountability will help you maintain the drive that will lead you to your best self. Holding yourself accountable is a way of self-respect because it bestows trust in yourself. When creating the parameters for accountability, it is important to set your goals. Goals are a way to be very specific about what you want to achieve, how, and when. It is easier to reach a goal when you are very clear about what it is and how you are going to get there. It is also very helpful in setting time frames. This way you can check on yourself, and you can ask others to check up on you, to help hold you accountable and keep you on track. In Chapter Seven, I will show you how to create specific goals as part of this program.

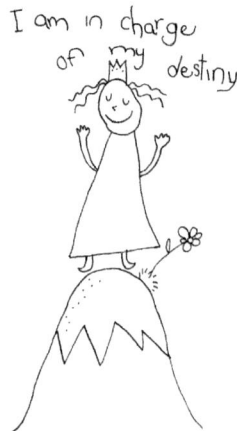

Part Three

THE RADIANT ENERGY PROGRAM

At this point I hope you have a better understanding of the mechanisms that rule the stress response and why supporting the HPA axis is so important. You should not be a helpless victim to chronic stress. You are not destined to a stressful daily grind devoid of luster and health. Being a mom does not equate to loss of vitality and glow. I am tired of being told motherhood is just stressful and that there is not much I can do about it. I refuse to believe that. I want radiant health. I want glowing skin. I want a life filled with purpose and joy. And I want all that for you too.

This is why I designed the Radiant Energy program. It is an educational resource designed to assist you in learning how to reduce stress and create habits that support balance in your body. The program focuses on reducing stressors and providing you with the tools you need to deal with them. Every week you will focus on a crucial aspect to support happy hormones. Sleep, detoxification, and nourishment will become your mantra. These backbones of wellness will lay the foundation to your health transformation. The program is an alternative to the conventional approach to stress, which mostly relies on sleeping pills, anti-depressants, prescription drugs, and antihistamines to deal with fatigue, anxiety, and poor overall health. It presents an opportunity to sustain health by creating balance in the body. By re-establishing restful sleep, reducing inflammation through detoxification, and providing the body with the nutrients it needs to perform optimally, you can enjoy motherhood in health. By following the recommended practices and creating habits, you can expect to see improvement in your energy levels, mood, skin and overall health.

There are few things as powerful as empowered women. Healthy, confident, and vibrant women can change the tide of the stress health epidemic and create a ripple effect that will have an impact on our children for generations to come.

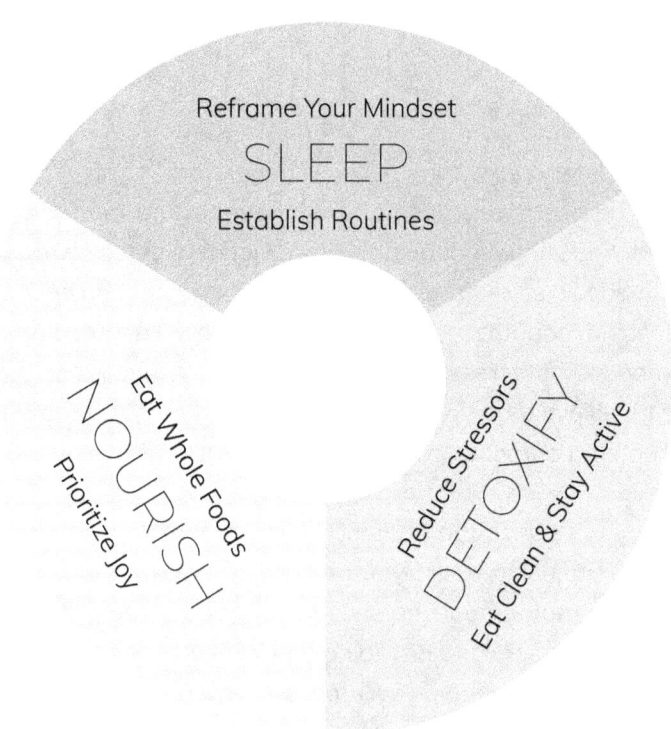

Chapter Seven

SETTING UP GOALS

Defining goals and intentions is an integral component of taking charge of your actions and reactions.[61] Research shows that people who write down their goals and share them are, on average, 33 percent more successful in accomplishing them than those who merely formulate goals.[62] To give yourself the best chance at success with this program, set aside a few minutes to write down your goals.

Make sure your goals are clear and reasonable. Vague goals are harder to achieve because it might be difficult to determine what it is you want – not to mention they don't give you any guidelines as to how or when you will achieve said goal. Goals that are too ambitious might work for some, but they will also set expectations too high. This might prove discouraging if the goal is not achieved in a reasonable time frame.

Before setting your goals, take a quick look at the basics of the program in the following chapters. This will help you figure out what goals are realistic for you at this time. Think about where you are right now and what it would take for you to complete this program to your satisfaction. If you are up to the challenge of completing the program in three weeks, take that into account. When planning to complete the program in three weeks, I advise you to set individual goals for each week; achieving smaller goals in a short amount of time will inspire you to keep going. So at the beginning of each week, write your goal or goals for that specific week. If you feel like you would need more than three weeks to complete the program, think of a time frame that you feel comfortable with and adjust your goals accordingly. Try not to make it too long though, because it will lead to procrastination. Procrastination is not your best friend when you are trying to create meaningful change.

When writing down your goal or goals, keep the SMART acronym in mind.

- **S**pecific. Be clear about what you wish to achieve, why is it important, and how you plan to do it.
- **M**easurable. There should be a quantifiable way to note where you are in the process of achieving your goal. This will help you stay motivated and on track.
- **A**chievable. Don't go too crazy. Think of what is possible for you right now. Keep it challenging and exciting but not unrealistic.
- **R**elevant. Make sure the goal or goals are important to you and that they align with your life.
- **T**ime specific. Set up a time frame for when you will begin and when you will finish. Give your goal a target date and work your way towards it.

A SMART goal will sound something like this: "I am creating a schedule in order to introduce one new habit every other day for one week. I will stay open and flexible. At the end of the week, I will have introduced three healthy habits that will support balance in my body."

Once you have written down your goal or goals, place that paper on your fridge, mirror or any place you can see it daily.

Are you ready to transform your health? Let's do it!

Chapter Eight

WEEK ONE: RESTORE SLEEP

Sleep is non-negotiable when it comes to health, and so, as most moms are notoriously sleep deprived, we will start here.

Insufficient sleep is associated with poor mood, fatigue, obesity, dull skin, premature aging, and the development of chronic disease. Motherhood can be draining, but there is no reason to give up on sleep. You can restore your radiance and vitality by creating habits that support restful sleep.

Step One: Set Up Your Bedroom

Your bedroom environment has a great impact on your sleep. Create a space that reflects your most peaceful self. With a few adjustments, you can optimize your bedroom and your sleep.

1. Declutter.

Your bedroom is a place for sleep or romance; it is not the garage. Try to remove sources of distraction like screens and trinkets. Keep it clean, simple, and comfortable.

2. Keep it dark.

As I explained earlier, the circadian rhythm is ruled by the dark/light cycle. Artificial light can mimic natural light, preventing your body from getting ready for sleep. Cell phones, screens, and night lights should all be removed at bedtime. I recommend using a blackout sleeping mask. Blackout curtains can also be a great investment.

3. Keep it cool.

As your body prepares to sleep, your temperature drops. Keeping your room cool can support sleep. The recommended room temperature for sleep is between 60 and 67 degrees Fahrenheit.

4. Keep it quiet.

Sudden noises are like sleep thieves. Along with keeping TVs or other entertainment systems out of the bedroom, a noise-canceling machine could be helpful for those noises we have no control over. I recommend using earplugs as an inexpensive alternative to keep noise to a minimum every night. If you have a baby and can't completely shut down, I recommend taking turns with your partner so some nights you are responsible for waking with the baby and some nights they are.

5. Try aromatherapy.

Studies have shown that aromatherapy can be effective in the improvement of mothers' sleep quality.[63] Lavender has been studied for its effects on the autonomic nervous system with positive results.[64] Diffusing essential oils like lavender, chamomile, and ylang-ylang can help induce your mind to a state conducive to sleep.

Step Two: Establish a Bedtime Routine

Consistency is without a doubt an incredibly influential tool in your wellness arsenal. One of the most powerful things I did as a new mom was to establish a consistent bedtime routine for my baby, well, as consistent as you can be with a night creature. Studies suggest that introducing a consistent nightly bedtime routine helps improve numerous aspects of infant and toddler sleep, like wakefulness after sleep onset and sleep continuity.[65] It also helps improve maternal mood. I have tested this theory with great success. I would always do bath, feeding, rocking/reading, and bedtime starting at the same time every night. As my babies grew, I kept basically the same routine. I am elated to report that to this day my 9 and 6 year old are in bed by 7:30pm, allowing my husband and me to have some time to unwind and connect before we go to bed. Consistent bedtime routines are not just wonderful for your kids; they are health promoting for you too. Creating a bedtime routine that works for you will prove invaluable to your wellness goals. Dedicate 30 minutes before bed to a relaxing ritual that will set you up to get the most restorative sleep possible. Screens off during that time too; it is an opportunity to soothe your mind. Meditation, breathing exercises, aromatherapy, a mini facial, or massage are all good ways to unwind. Start your daily bedtime ritual as close to 9:30 p.m. as possible so you can be in bed by 10:00 p.m.

As part of your bedtime routine, you can use any of the following relaxation exercises.

Relaxing Breath

Place the tip of your tongue just behind your upper front teeth, and keep it there while you do this exercise. Close your mouth, and inhale through your nose to the count of four. Hold your breath for a count of seven. Exhale through your mouth, making a whoosh sound to a count of eight. Repeat this cycle three more times.

One Minute Meditation

- Sit comfortably. Close your eyes.
- Take three deep belly breaths in and out.
- On the next breath say silently to yourself or out loud:

- "Head relax."
- On the next one:
- "Eyes relax."
- With every breath, you will ask your body to relax.
- "Nose relax."
- "Ears relax."
- "Mouth relax."
- "Chin relax."
- "Shoulders relax."
- "Chest relax."
- "Belly relax."
- "Arms relax."
- "Hands relax."
- "Fingers relax."
- "Hips relax."
- "Legs relax."
- "Feet relax."
- "Toes relax."
- Take one more deep belly breath in and out. Say "Thank you."

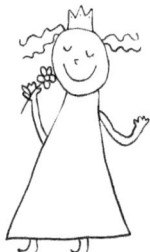

Mini Facial Massage

Begin by using the tips of your index and middle fingers and make small circles under and around each eye. Continue making small circles around the forehead, cheekbones, and down the sides of the jaw and chin. Continue with small circles for several moments. When done, relax hands and take three slow, deep breaths.

> Tip: Use this massage when applying your moisturizer or serum.

> Anytime you are getting stressed or tense, stop for a second and acknowledge your feelings. Take one to three deep breaths, and let the tension go. Re-center yourself, and start over or continue what you were doing.

Step Three: Time Your Meals

Meal timing is linked to sleep through genes that control energy balance.[66] New research from the MRC Laboratory of Molecular Biology in Cambridge and the University of Manchester found that meal timing influences your internal clock, which controls the sleep/wake cycles, via insulin.[67] This hormone was identified as a primary signal that relates the timing of meals to the cellular clocks across our body. For example, skipping breakfast disrupts our internal clock by altering the activity of enzymes, hormones, and transport systems that control different aspects of metabolism.[68] This leads to poor energy and spikes in blood sugar levels when we finally eat.

Imagine your body is a factory. The factory machines are at full swing during the hours of 6 a.m. till 6 p.m. producing energy. At 6 p.m., the machines shut down, and the machine operators leave. At this time, the maintenance crews show up to clean and repair the machines. This part of the operation can only occur between 6 p.m. and 6 a.m. Now imagine that the day shift workers start showing up late and staying past 6 p.m. If the day shift workers constantly stay overtime eventually the machines would start malfunctioning because the maintenance crew would be left with little time to care for the machines.

The times we eat can determine what time which workers show up. So, if you are skipping breakfast and having late dinners on a regular basis, you are sending the wrong workers at the wrong times, promoting the detriment of the machines and minimizing the efficiency of the factory that is your body.

Eat your meals at consistent times this week. Have breakfast within two hours of waking, and space your meals to have roughly four to four and a half hours in between. For example: breakfast at 9:00 a.m., lunch at 1:30 p.m. and dinner around 5:30-6:00 p.m. Feel free to have snacks that are low in sugar and high in protein between meals. Sweetened beverages, caffeine, and alcohol should be avoided or strictly limited, especially after 4:00 p.m. In order to get your body ready for restful sleep, have dinner before 8 p.m. and avoid foods that are high in fat and low in fiber. If you need a snack before bed, choose one from the "mellow out" section on the snack suggestion chart found in Chapter Eleven.

During this week, I encourage you to prepare the Magic Mineral Broth by Rebecca Katz. Its high mineral content makes it a perfect pre-bedtime tea. This recipe is easy to prepare and will begin the healing process. I use this recipe all the time. I give it to my kids regularly, especially during the flu season. You can find the recipe on page 122.

PRODUCE	PROTEIN	OTHER
Spinach	Shrimp	Raw Honey
Spring Salad	Cod	Oatmeal
Bell Peppers	Tuna	Plain Whole Yogurt
Cremini Mushrooms	Chicken	Feta Cheese
Avocado	Turkey	Chamomile Tea
Bananas	Tofu	Pumpkin Seeds
Berries	Eggs	Flax Seeds
Melons	Pinto Beans	Sunflower Seeds
Cherries		
Kiwi		

The foods on this chart contain nutrients like magnesium, potassium, tryptophan, omega 3s, antioxidants, and b-vitamins, which help promote relaxation.

Step Four: Balance Light Exposure

Sleep is heavily influenced by light and darkness. One of the easiest ways to balance your circadian rhythm is to follow the natural cycles of the day, particularly in the morning.[69] Make it a habit to wake up at the same time every morning. When you wake up, make sure to get some light exposure as quickly as possible. Light signals travel from your eyes to your brain and let it know it is time to start daytime activities. You can stand by a window or have your morning tea outside. During the day, go for a walk and spend time outside. In colder months, or if you spend a lot of time in the office, use a light therapy lamp. I use one regularly. It does not need to be expensive, mine was under $30. At night, make sure your bedroom is dark, and remove electronics if possible. Avoiding screen time before bed, as I've recommended for your bedtime routine, is best, but if you must use screens, try wearing blue light filtration glasses. Some studies show they could be beneficial in treating insomnia.[70,71]

Scheduled exposure to light and darkness will help improve your energy, mood, and sleep patterns.

Step Five: Practice Gratitude

Studies show that gratitude is associated with better sleep, reduced anxiety, and better mood. A positive mindset is key to health, and it begins with gratitude. Being grateful creates a ripple effect that will help you sleep and feel better.

Your two gratitude assignments for this week are:

1. Say "thank you" every morning when you wake and before you put your feet on the ground.

2. Before going to bed every night, write three to five things you were grateful for that day in your gratitude notebook.

Checklist WEEK ONE

- [ ] Peaceful Bedroom
  - [ ] Declutter
  - [ ] Dark
  - [ ] Cool
  - [ ] Quiet
  - [ ] Aromatherapy
- [ ] Bedtime Routine
  - [ ] Screens off 30 minutes before bed
  - [ ] Bedtime rituals
- [ ] Positive Affirmations
- [ ] Gratitude Journal
- [ ] Timed Meals
- [ ] Morning Exposure to Daylight
- [ ] Afternoon Exposure to Daylight
- [ ] Self-Love

Chapter Nine

WEEK TWO: DETOXIFICATION

Detoxification is the process of reducing or eliminating a toxic compound. In our bodies this is achieved through chemical processes that render the toxic materials less toxic so they can be expelled.[72] There are numerous routes for detoxification in our bodies. Our liver, lungs, skin, lymphatic system, gut, kidneys, and brain all work together to maintain equilibrium. Our body is prepared to detoxify when needed, which is every day. But if we overburden it with toxicity, detoxification pathways become impaired. Symptoms that could point to problems with detoxification include brain fog, fatigue, unhealthy skin, allergies, food sensitivities, poor mood, premature aging, unstable weight, infertility, and low libido.[73] You might be thinking these symptoms are very similar to those of HPA axis dysfunction, and you would be correct. That is because these systems work together. HPA axis dysfunction will create inflammation in the body, and this will increase your toxic burden. Excess toxicity will cause more stress. All this stress will overstimulate HPA axis function and another destructive cycle begins. If the stressor is not dealt with, the stress response will be on a never-ending loop, causing toxicity, inflammation and more stress.

Just like the rest of your body systems, detoxification systems work in and for balance. Our bodies work as a united front. If one system becomes impaired, the rest will follow.

Step One: Reduce Toxic Foods

Foods can provide us with the nutrients our body needs to perform all its functions. But some foods do the opposite: they take away nutrients or block nutrient absorption in our bodies. Added sugars, damaged fats (like those found in fried foods), and overly refined and processed foods rob our bodies of nutrients and promote inflammation. This creates a toxic environment in our bodies, making us more susceptible to disease and allergies. These foods serve no nutritional purpose but they use up energy and our nutrient reserves. This week you will focus on avoiding added sugars entirely. While this will be our main goal, I suggest you take a look at the sidebar listing foods to avoid and consider eliminating them from your diet at some point.

Foods to avoid:

Damaged fats, like refined vegetable oils, and trans fats. You will find these in baked goods, fried foods, and many prepackaged snacks.

Foods treated with pesticides. Conventionally grown produce can be loaded with toxic pesticides. Always wash your produce before consuming. The best way to avoid pesticides is by choosing organic produce when possible.

Animal products high in hormones and antibiotics. Factory farmed animals are often pumped full of hormones and antibiotics; these inevitably end up in their muscle and fat tissue. Try to always choose organic animal products. For more information on animal product labeling visit the environmental working group. You can use this link to access information of labeling https://www.ewg.org/research/labeldecoder/

Fast foods. These convenient and popular foods are extremely nutrient deficient and often made with cheap and dubious ingredients. They are high in damaged fats, additives, food colorings and preservatives.

Overly refined foods. The term edible food like substances, made popular by food journalist Michael Pollan, refers to foods that are mostly made in a lab. These types of foods contain many chemicals that are harmful to our bodies. Some examples: breakfast bars/substitutes, cheese-like products (American cheese slices, liquid cheese, powdered cheese, etc), portable yogurts in tubes, and protein bars. If the ingredient list is long and you can barely pronounce the ingredients in it, avoid it.

Eliminating Added Sugars

Added sugars are those that do not occur naturally in foods. When sugars are placed in foods to add or intensify flavor they are considered added sugars. They are anti-nutrients because they have no nutritional value. They use up nutrient stores in the body, and they can block nutrient absorption. They are associated with obesity, diabetes, heart disease, poor immune function, and rapid aging. Avoiding added sugars completely for a week is a great way to help reset your overall wellness. This is **not** an in-depth sugar detox, so you shouldn't experience great discomfort. The benefits of eliminating added sugars increase with time. Doing this for one week will give you a boost and inspire you to do it longer for more profound results.

For now, let's focus on getting through this week.

Guidelines

Learn to identify sugars and their many names. Added sugars are in 74 percent of packaged foods, hidden under many aliases and can be found in many prepackaged foods. Keep an eye on sauces, ketchup, bread, and salad dressings as they often contain added sugars.

Here are some alternate names for added sugar. Look for these on ingredient labels so you know what you are getting:

Agave nectar
Barbados sugar
Barley
Malt-barley
Malt syrup
Beet sugar
Brown sugar
Buttered syrup
Cane juice
Cane juice crystals
Cane sugar
Caramel
Carob syrup
Castor sugar
Coconut palm sugar
Coconut sugar
Confectioners' sugar
Corn sweetener
Corn syrup
Corn syrup solids
Date sugar

Dehydrated cane juice
Demerara sugar
Dextrin
Dextrose
Evaporated cane juice
Free-flowing brown sugars
Fructose
Fruit juice
Fruit juice concentrate
Glucose
Glucose solids
Golden sugar
Golden syrup
Grape sugar
Hfcs (high-fructose corn syrup)
Honey
Icing sugar
Invert sugar
Malt syrup

Maltodextrin
Maltol
Maltose
Mannose
Maple syrup
Molasses
Muscovado
Palm sugar
Panocha
Powdered sugar
Raw sugar
Refiner's syrup
Rice syrup
Saccharose
Sorghum
Syrup
Sucrose
Sugar (granulated)
Sweet sorghum Syrup
Treacle-turbinado sugar
Yellow sugar

Sugars found in whole fruits, vegetables, and milk are okay. Homemade, unsweetened vegetable or fruit smoothies are okay too. Prepare your meals and snacks at home. If eating out, remember desserts, sweet condiments, juices, sodas, and cocktails contain added sugars.

Processed/pre-packaged foods containing sugars are to be avoided. Avoid table sugars, syrups, honey, and artificial sweeteners. Prepackaged and refined food products like flavored milk, yogurts, granola bars, cereals, and juices contain added sugars. Even products labeled as "healthy" can contain high amounts of sugar. Do not be fooled by labels that say all-natural, no artificial sweeteners, fat-free, low fat, or heart-healthy. There is very little regulation when it comes to making health claims, so even foods that claim to be good for you are usually not. For example, if a breakfast bar claims to give you four hours of nutritious steady energy, yet it contains 13 grams of added sugars per serving, it is more likely to create a sugar rush that will not provide you with a steady source of energy. Always look at the food/nutrition label and list of ingredients, not at the "health" claims on the front label.

HOW TO FIND SUGAR IN A SUGAR LABEL

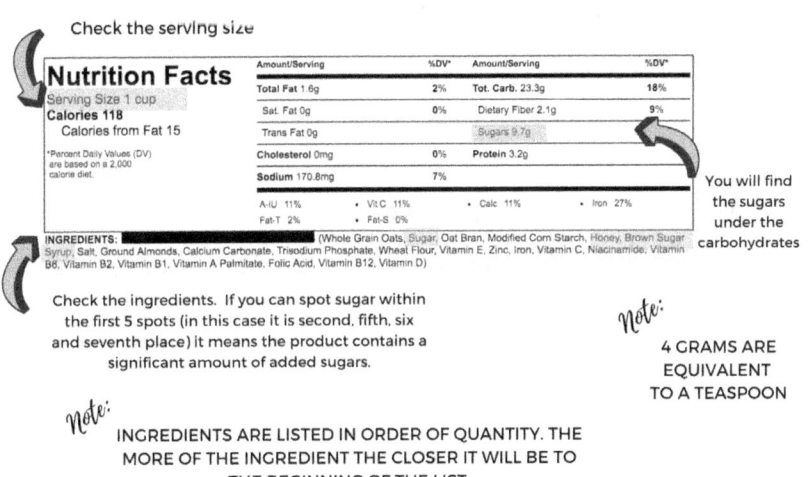

Stay with it. It is only one week, and you can do it!

Key Points About Sugar

1. To make their products seem healthier, manufacturers use smaller amounts of many types of sugars in a single product. This doesn't mean the product is low in sugars. Always look at the ingredients.

2. Swapping sucrose for natural or "healthy" sugars does not make a product high in sugar healthier. Agave, honey, maple syrup, and coconut sugar are still sugars and should be consumed sparingly.

3. Keep an eye on portion size. What you might consider a serving might be more than one.

4. Manufacturers will print lots of health claims, making products seem healthy when they're really full of added sugar. Always read the nutrition label.

5. The detrimental health effects of a diet high in sugars have been well documented. If you want balanced hormones, healthy skin, vibrant energy, and a strong immune system, keep sugars at bay. The American Heart Association's recommendation is to limit your added sugar intake to less than 10 percent of your daily caloric intake.

6. For optimal health or if you are struggling with obesity or chronic disease, I would suggest keeping your added sugars under 5 percent of your daily caloric intake. That's roughly 12.5 grams for women, 19 grams for men and 6-12.5 grams for children.

I recommend including a cup of turmeric tea every day this week to assist with detoxification. You can also try any of the beverages that support detoxification. See beverage recipes starting on page 122

Step Two: Reduce Your Toxic Load

Toxicity cannot be avoided completely. Every day we are exposed to hundreds of chemicals. Hormone-disrupting chemicals can be found in the air we breathe, the food we eat, the water we drink, and the products we put on our skin. Even our bodies produce toxins as by-products of metabolism and detoxification. The best we can do is try to avoid some chemicals and support detoxification so our body has the best chance at maintaining balance and health. Use the following suggestions to reduce your toxic load.

Personal Care Products

- Most products you find in the beauty aisle are loaded with hormone disruptors. While it is difficult to avoid all harmful chemicals, staying informed and shopping mindfully can help lower your exposure to them.
- The Environmental Working Group's Skin Deep database can help you select safer alternatives: https://www.ewg.org/skindeep/
- Avoid products that contain parabens, formaldehyde, phthalates, aluminum, sodium laureth sulfate, propylene glycol, hydroquinone, alcohol, mineral oil, petrolatum, talc, artificial dyes, and synthetic fragrances.

Household Products

- When buying home cleaning products and detergents, look for those that are not petroleum based and are free of phosphates and chlorine.
- Unless derived from natural essential oils, do not use products that contain "fragrance" in their ingredient list.
- If you have a little extra time, you can make your own household cleaning products. There are many free recipes online. The

Environmental Working Group has a free guide with recipes. You can use this link: https://cdn3.ewg.org/sites/default/files/u352/EWG_SpringCleaningGuide.pdf
- If you have less time, you can choose products from the many brands that offer natural cleaning products. Visit the EWG Home Guide to help you find cleaner solutions for your home: https://www.ewg.org/healthyhomeguide/

Stress

- If under a lot of stress, consider using a vitamin B complex supplement. Use as directed on the bottle.
- Massage. If your budget allows it, get a professional one. It is a fabulous way to support your lymphatic system. Along with helping you relax, it will also help you detox.
- Create a relaxing playlist. Select from instrumental songs created for relaxation. These are easy to find on almost all music subscription channels or free on YouTube. Use headphones and close your eyes for a more intense experience.
- Pay attention to your breathing. Every hour try to take three to five deep belly breaths.
- Avoid toxic people, toxic media, and toxic thoughts.

Pampering For Detoxification

Jade Roller

Use a jade roller to give yourself a mini face massage. It helps stimulate collagen production and detoxification. You can also use your jade roller to apply your favorite clean moisturizer. This will help increase absorption.

Dry Brushing

Dry brushing is a great way to support detoxification. Some of the benefits are exfoliation, stimulating circulation, and supporting lymph drainage.

Bentonite Clay
Bentonite clay is rich in minerals and helps draw out toxins from the body. It makes for a fantastic pore reducing mask that can help nourish your skin. Just mix a spoonful with a little water and apply to face and neck. Leave on for 10 minutes or until dry, and then remove with a damp towel or warm water.

Epsom Salts
Epsom salts are rich in magnesium. An Epsom salt bath is not only supportive of detoxification, but it also promotes relaxation, pain relief, and helps reduce inflammation. Dissolve a cup in a warm bath, and add a few drops of your favorite essential oil for an invigorating or soothing experience. I like to add a cup of coconut milk for a moisturizing and luxurious bath.

Step Three: Be Mindful

Health is not only based on the foods we eat. Health has everything to do with the way we treat ourselves, the company we keep, the relationships we nurture, and the thoughts we allow in our daily lives. After detoxing from unhealthy foods and chemical-laden house and beauty products, we should examine other sources of toxicity in our lives. Toxic relationships, jobs, ignoring traumatic experiences, and inner chatter are very damaging to our health. This week, examine the people, noise, and activities you surround yourself with, and think about ways to distance yourself from those that harm you. Allow yourself to feel whatever it is you are feeling now, and explore ways to heal. Pay attention to the way you speak to and treat yourself. Be kind and patient with yourself. Try to maintain your focus on what is in front of you to avoid getting stuck in past situations or worrying about possible outcomes. The past is over, and the future is not here yet; you are here now. Practice loving this moment.

Step Four: Hydrate

Clean water is crucial for flushing out toxins from the body. Sugary beverages, alcohol, and coffee are dehydrating and they can add to the body's toxic load. Aiming to consume half your body weight (measured in pounds) in ounces of water daily is a simple step you can take to support the detoxification process. For example, if you weigh 160 pounds, aim to drink 80 ounces of water a day. If you are consuming lots of fruits and vegetables, the amount of water needed can be reduced as you will absorb it from those foods. Remember, this is an estimate, as your body's water needs will vary with age, health condition, weight, activity level, and weather. Pay attention to your body. Thirst, dark yellow urine, cramps, fatigue, irritability, headaches, and dry eyes, mouth or skin, can all be signs of dehydration.

Step Five: Exercise

There is no pill that will give you the benefits of an enjoyable routine exercise program. Finding your dream workout is part of your journey to health, and its benefits are countless. Toxin removal, increased blood flow, endurance, strength, bone health, mental health, radiant skin, elevated mood, weight loss or maintenance, and increased energy are just a few of the benefits of a regular workout.[74] This week try working out for a minimum of 30 minutes for 3 days. If you can do more, even better. Use the following ideas for inspiration. Remember these are meant to motivate you to stay active; they are not the advice of a fitness expert. A workout should be suitable to your physical needs and health. To avoid physical injury, be mindful of your current health state, exercise in a way that is safe for you, and consult your doctor or fitness expert if you are not sure if a workout is right for you.

Walk

Including a 30-minute walk in your routine is an amazing strategy to create health. It can help with weight loss, improve cardiovascular fitness, boost energy, strengthen bones, and improve mood. Walking will also give you a chance to connect with nature, to be outside, and to get some sunshine to support your circadian rhythm.

Yoga

Muscle tone and strength, improved respiration and vitality, flexibility, and balance are just a few of the benefits of a yoga practice. It is a gentle yet powerful workout that helps restore balance and health. Try it at home or at a local studio.

Play With the Kids

An often overlooked method of working out is performing physical activities with your kids. Throwing a frisbee, hula hooping, or playing tag are ways to exercise. Try the Animal Workout:

Get down on all fours and walk in a circle like different animals. You can be agile like a cat, slow like a turtle, big like an elephant, or silly like a monkey. It is not only a great way to get moving, but a fun way to bond with the kids.

Dance

From improved coordination to better memory, the benefits of dancing are numerous. It can be done as a high intensity or aerobic workout. Zumba, salsa, ballroom dancing, and barre classes are just a few examples of the many ways that you can incorporate dance into your life. If you are not ready to go out in public, you can try one of the many free instructional videos on YouTube or any of your streaming subscriptions.

HIIT Workout

If you are looking for something more intense and less time consuming, a high-intensity interval training (HIIT) workout might be right for you. HIIT workouts are done in short but intense bouts, followed by periods of resting. One of the cool things about HIIT workouts is that your body continues to burn calories after you are done.[75]

This type of workout is better done under the supervision of a trained professional. If you are fit for it, it packs a lot of reward in a small period of time.

Checklist WEEK TWO

- [ ] Avoid Added Sugars
- [ ] Avoid Damaged Fats
  - [ ] Fried and pre-packaged foods
- [ ] Hydrate
  - [ ] Half your body weight in ounces of water
- [ ] Reduced Toxic Load
  - [ ] Organic foods
  - [ ] Clean beauty and personal care products
  - [ ] Toxin-free house cleaning products
  - [ ] Relaxation rituals
- [ ] Detoxing Beverages
- [ ] Detoxification Rituals
- [ ] Exercising
- [ ] Self-love

Chapter Ten

WEEK THREE: NOURISHMENT

Once your body has gone through detoxification, the healing begins. During this time, it is very important to give your body the nutrients and care it needs to regain balance. Health is about balance. It is about making the choices that will support your body, mind, and spirit. It is about habits, consistency, knowledge, and lots of love. This week is all about nourishing your body with good food, good relationships, and good times. Have fun, and remember, you deserve the best!

Step One: Eat Colorfully

Foods work in a synergetic way. Nutrients require the help of other nutrients to function optimally. The best way to get the most out of your meals is to eat a variety of whole foods. Fruits and vegetables are nutrition powerhouses. They contain vitamins, minerals, carbohydrates, protein, fats, and unmatched antioxidant power. This week's focus is on including a variety of fruits and vegetables in every meal. Make sure to include them in your breakfast, lunch, and dinner. Check out the Menu Planner at the end of this chapter for some ideas.

> Try the healing cinnamon and chamomile tea. See recipe on page 125.

Step Two: Include Lots of Leafy Greens

Dark, leafy greens are an incredible source of anti-aging nutrients. Studies show their powerful effect on cognitive function, as well as macular, cardiac, bone, and skin health.[76-78] This week have at least one cup of, or a combination of the following every day: spinach, collard greens, cabbage, kale, arugula, or chard. They are nutrient dense and very low in calories. You can have them at breakfast, lunch, or dinner.

In addition to the cup of greens, try to include a salad with dinner every night. This is an easy way to increase your vegetable intake and help reduce acidity in the body. If you buy a salad mix, it can be as simple as adding a handful to your plate. I recommend always having a big bowl of salad on the table during dinner time. Making this a habit will help everyone in the family get used to consuming leafy greens instead of thinking of it as an oddity.

> Chewing your food well is the first step to digestive health. If your body cannot digest food properly, it cannot absorb its nutrients. Chew your food thoroughly, until almost liquid, before swallowing. Eating in a calm, mindful way will not only improve your dining experience, it will enhance digestion.

Step Three: Supplement

A balanced diet based on whole foods is the best way to obtain most of the nutrients your body needs. Unfortunately, even those eating a balanced diet will often find themselves short. Some people believe you can get all the nutrients you need from food. In my opinion, this piece of advice is misguided and misleading. While nutrients are better when coming from whole foods, most foods lack nutrients, and few people eat a diet that consistently delivers the nutrients required for optimal health. Poor soil quality has decreased the nutrient content of our foods.[79] People suffering from any form of disease, including stress, often require higher amounts of nutritional support. And let's face it, the standard American diet is not only nutrient deficient, it is nutrient depleting. For these reasons, I believe professional grade supplements can be of great value for optimal health.

How to Select Your Supplements

- Check the ingredients list and avoid supplements that contain binders, fillers, inactive substances, lubricants, colorants, sweeteners, flavorings, and coating materials. These are usually found in low-quality supplements. Purchasing a poor quality supplement is usually a waste of money, no matter how cheap it is.
- Most nutrients are better absorbed in natural vs. synthetic form. Try to select supplements that are derived from a natural source and made with non-genetically modified organism (GMO) ingredients.
- Check the label for the Good Manufacturing Practices (GMP) compliant seal.
- Check that the supplement's facts label establishes the quantities of each ingredient.
- Higher quality supplements will usually have a full description on the back of the label of ingredients, including the sources that are used in the manufacturing of the product. A generic health claim like "Vitamin C is a powerful antioxidant" or "This multivitamin has all the nutrients you need" is not sufficient.
- A good company will usually have a website loaded with information about their product, scientific research, educational resources, and dedicate a portion of their proceeds to further research.

Recommended Supplements

Multivitamin with Mineral Complex

Choose one that requires more than one serving a day, such as two tablets twice a day, for example. This helps with the size of the tablet and with spreading nutrient doses throughout the day. Take them at separate times; I recommend breakfast and lunch.

D3

The amount of vitamin D required for optimal health will vary according to age, weight, health status, sun exposure, and diet. According to the National Institutes of Health, a dose of up to 4,000 IU (international units) of vitamin D is safe for anyone older than 9 years. Because vitamin D deficiencies are very common, and the standard American diet and lifestyle promote these deficiencies, I highly encourage using a supplement. Try to get it in liquid form or gel capsule. Research suggests it is better absorbed in an oil vehicle.[80] You can use what is suggested on the bottle or consult with your health practitioner of choice.

Complement your supplement with food sources of vitamin D.

Food Sources of Vitamin D

Oily fish like salmon	about 149 IU per ounce
Shiitake mushrooms	about 3 IU per piece
Cod liver oil	about 1,360 IU per tablespoon
Egg yolk	about 260 IU per serving
Meat	about 9 IU per 3 oz serving
Dairy products	about 102 IU per cup

Omega-3 Fats

Select a high-potency supplement containing at least 1,000 milligrams per serving. The supplement should include both EPA and DHA in triglyceride molecular form; you can check this on the label. Omega-3 fats are very delicate. Supplements should come from a brand that guarantees purity, stability and freshness.

Supplements work best when taken consistently. Keep this in mind, and make it part of your routine.

Step Four: Explore Food Sensitivities

Food sensitivities are different from food allergies (like nut allergies) or food intolerances (like lactose intolerance). Food sensitivities refer to a person's negative digestive reaction to a specific food. Unlike allergies, the symptoms or reactions take longer to present. Common reactions brought on by food sensitivities are stuffy nose, fatigue, mental fog, digestive problems, bloating, fluid retention, mood swings, and drowsiness. If you suffer from any of these symptoms on a regular basis, take note of the foods you consume. Some of the most problematic are gluten (a protein found in grains), dairy products, corn, nuts, eggs, shellfish, beef, pork, soy, and food additives (for example, artificial colors and nitrites). If you are not sure if you suffer from specific food sensitivities, a short term elimination diet would help you explore this. This is what you do. First eliminate a specific food for a minimum of two weeks. Then, notice if your symptoms subside. Finally, reintroduce the food gradually and take note if your symptoms show up again.

If you try an elimination diet and continue experiencing symptoms, you might be suffering from an autoimmune disease, such as celiac disease, which prevents your body from processing gluten. In this case you will need to be diagnosed by a health care practitioner and follow a strict diet. To explore this topic in more detail you can visit

the Food Allergy Research & Education organization's website at
https://www.foodallergy.org/

If you feel like you don't have the patience or time to do an elimination diet you can try an at home food sensitivity test. You can do a quick online search for food sensitivity tests to compare your options. Exploring food sensitivities could be a turning point for your diet and health.

Step Five: Do One Thing You Love That is Only for You

Taking care of ourselves is just as important as taking care of our children. We also deserve the best, and you are the only one that can give yourself the best. This week and every week from now on, make time to do one thing you love. Put it on the calendar, make a date with yourself and keep it. Make a promise to yourself to stop with the excuses, place yourself high on your to-do list and treat yourself with the same fierce and relentless love you treat your loved ones. This is the most powerful thing you can do for your health. Your well-being depends on this.

Checklist WEEK THREE

- [ ] Peaceful Bedroom
- [ ] Bedtime Routine
- [ ] Positive Affirmations
- [ ] Gratitude Journaling
- [ ] Nutrient Rich Diet
- [ ] Half Your Body Weight in Ounces of Water
- [ ] Getting Sunshine
- [ ] Fewer Sugars
- [ ] Active/Exercise
- [ ] Reduced Toxic Load
- [ ] Making Time for the Things I Love
- [ ] Relaxation Exercises
- [ ] Taking Supplements
- [ ] Self-love

Chapter Eleven
MENU PLANNING

The word diet is often given a negative tone in our culture. For example, you might hear a friend say: "I am on a diet so I cannot eat anything I like." It has become the antagonizing villain in every woman's mission of reaching her health and weight goals. I would like you to break up with that stereotype. The word diet simply refers to the foods you eat habitually. That is all. From now on I would like you to think of your diet as the way you nourish your body, not as a trend you must obsess over or guilt yourself into.

The food recommendations in this menu plan are meant to support you and your body.

VEGETARIAN PROTEIN SOURCES

Lentils: 18 grams of protein per cup
Chia Seeds: 2 grams of protein per tablespoon
Tempeh: 30.8 grams of protein per cup
Quinoa: 8 grams of protein per ¼ cup
Chickpeas: 9 grams of protein per ¼ cup
Cottage Cheese: 21.9 grams of protein per cup
Spirulina: 4.02 grams of protein per tablespoon
Green Peas: 7.9 grams of protein per cup

Breakfast

Steps for a Balancing Breakfast:

1. Have breakfast within two hours of waking up.
2. Include fiber from fruits, vegetables, nuts, or whole grains.
3. Include healthy fats from nuts, avocados, seeds, coconut oil, good quality organic butter, or ghee (clarified butter).
4. Include protein from nuts, eggs, whole grains, or good quality animal protein. Aim for at least 15 grams.
5. Eat mindfully and chew your food thoroughly.

While you sleep, your body is fasting. When you awake, your body needs to break that fast in order to produce the energy it needs to start your daily activities. Having a breakfast containing protein and healthy fats will improve your meal satisfaction, appetite, and sleep quality. It will also encourage you to make healthier meal choices throughout the day.[81] A high-protein breakfast supports weight loss because it increases energy expenditure (burning calories), keeps your hunger-controlling hormones in check, helps regulate sugar levels in the blood, and increases muscle mass.[82] The amount of protein that is ideal for you will vary according to age, health status, activity level, weight, sex, and fitness goals. Aim for at least 15 grams of protein during breakfast. This could be two eggs and a spoonful of peanut butter, for example. You can use a protein calculator app or website, like calculator.net, to help you determine what is right for you. Aim to spread your protein intake throughout the day but make sure to have a good amount during breakfast. If you are vegetarian or would like to reduce your intake of animal protein, check out the vegetarian sources of protein sidebar. Do not skip breakfast, and avoid breakfasts that are high in refined carbohydrates, like cereal. Eating these will create a perfect storm for problems with insulin, promoting fatigue, disease, and weight gain. Breakfast is meant to increase energy levels in the morning and set the stage for your day, so make it count.

BREAKFAST MENU PLANNER
(See recipes starting on page 102.)

SUNDAY	Power Up Omelet Serve with a side of fresh fruit or in a bed of leafy greens.
MONDAY	Open faced turkey sandwich on whole grain that includes leafy greens, tomatoes, and onion
TUESDAY	Power Up Oatmeal
WEDNESDAY	Avocado and Eggs
THURSDAY	Breakfast Smoothie Have with a slice of whole grain toast with avocado on the side.
FRIDAY	Breakfast Burrito with scrambled eggs, avocado, feta cheese, and sauteed peppers, onions, mushrooms, and spinach
SATURDAY	Fruit Yogurt Cup with pumpkin seeds and flax seeds drizzled with honey

Lunch

Steps for an Energizing Lunch:

1. Have lunch about four hours after breakfast.
2. Include two vegetable servings (roughly the equivalent of one cup).
3. Include a source of protein like legumes or clean animal protein, about 15 grams.
4. Avoid sugary beverages and refined carbohydrates like pastries, breads, and pasta.
5. Eat mindfully and chew your food thoroughly.

If you make a habit of skipping or procrastinating lunch, it's time to change. Lunch is as important as breakfast because it will provide you with the energy you need to continue feeling energized. Keeping blood sugar levels stable throughout the day is one of the main components of a healthful diet. In order to support mood, energy, and healthy weight your body needs nutrients to fuel normal function. Do not ignore your body's cues, like the afternoon slump. Make a nourishing lunch part of your daily routine.

LUNCH MENU PLANNER
(See recipes starting on page 107).

SUNDAY	Omega-3 Power Salad
MONDAY	Zoodles and Chicken
TUESDAY	Roasted Carrot and Ginger Soup Have with a side of nuts and avocado.
WEDNESDAY	Better Nachos
THURSDAY	Lentil Salad
FRIDAY	Chicken and Kale Salad
SATURDAY	Tuna or chicken salad on a bed of greens or in a lettuce wrap

Dinner

Steps for a Dinner That Supports Restoration:

1. Have dinner before 8:00 p.m.
2. Have nutrient-rich foods, plenty of vegetables, and a smaller portion of protein and healthy fats.
3. Include foods containing tryptophan, like beans, turkey, fish, or nuts/seeds.
4. Avoid caffeine, sugars, damaged fats, and refined carbohydrates.
5. Eat mindfully and chew your food thoroughly.

Dinners do not need to be heavy. They should be nutrient-rich so that your body has the tools it needs to relax, prepare for detoxification, and regenerate during sleeping hours. Include vegetables in your dinner. Make about 75 percent of your plate veggies, and fill the other 25 percent with healthy fats and protein. Avoid dinners that are high in fats, refined carbohydrates, and sugars. Also avoid dinners that are low in fiber. Your body heals while you sleep. Evening meals should be easy to digest in order to promote the relaxation that prepares your body for restorative sleep.

Try these dinner ideas which can double up as a lunch.

DINNER MENU PLANNER
(See recipes starting on page 113.)

SUNDAY	Roasted Cod and Sweet Potatoes
MONDAY	Seared Shrimp and Pumpkin Soup
TUESDAY	Vegetarian Chili
WEDNESDAY	Salmon with Green Goddess Quinoa Bowl
THURSDAY	Vegetable Tofu and Stir Fry
FRIDAY	Roasted Carrot and Ginger Soup Have with an open faced turkey sandwich on whole grain
SATURDAY	Sautéed kale, peppers, and mushroom with protein of choice.

SIDENOTE: Don't forget the salad.

Snacks

Nutrient-rich snacks are a fantastic way to keep blood sugar levels stable. Use this guide to select snacks that will provide you with lots of energy during the daytime hours and snacks that will help your body wind down when it is time to relax.

MOM TIP

Get a set of snack containers and fill them with fresh fruits, veggies (snap peas are great for this), organic cheese, or a nut mix. Prepare them for you and the kids, and you will always have a healthy snack ready to go.

POWER UP	MELLOW OUT
Celery or apple slices with nut butter and honey	Banana with nut butter
Carrots and hummus	Cup of cherries
Guacamole and chips	Kiwi slices
Cashews, almonds, walnuts, chickpeas (roasted), pumpkin seeds, and raisins. Make a mix and store in mason jar. Have ¼-½ cup as a daytime snack.	Pumpkin, sunflower, and sesame seeds. Make a mix and store in a mason jar. Have ¼ cup if you need a nighttime snack.

Pre-Packaged Snacks

Most of these can be found as single servings and are a good option when you are on the run: popcorn, guacamole/mashed avocado, roasted chickpeas, mixed nuts, nut bars that are low in sugar (less than 5 grams per serving), hummus, grass fed jerky, roasted seaweed, kale chips, and crudité cups with dip.

Transitional Foods

Transitional foods are those that are used during the process of changing your diet from one that is high in refined foods to one that is based on whole foods. These foods serve as substitutions to nutrient-depleting foods you might consume on a regular basis. Some of the ingredients you will want to substitute include:

- Natural sources of sugars like those found in fruits, instead of added sugars
- Healthier and stable fats found in coconut or avocado oil, instead of the damaged fats found in fried food
- Naturally occurring colors, instead of artificial colors

Look for foods that are made with natural ingredients and that have a short ingredient list, where you can read and recognize all the ingredients. For example, if using peanut butter, make sure the only ingredients are peanuts and salt. Avoid foods that list a variety of sugars, artificial colors, artificial flavors, vegetable oils like canola or soybean, and preservatives you have trouble pronouncing. The ingredients in your foods should be recognizable to you.

Use transitional foods to reduce your exposure to damaging foods while slowly making the conversion to health-promoting foods. In the long run, some transitional foods can be eliminated or consumed occasionally.

Examples Of Transitional and Healthier Foods

Worst Choices	Better Choices
Regular potato chips	Organic potato chips baked in coconut oil
Chocolate candy bar	Nut bar or nuts with raisins and a few chocolate chips
Regular flavored yogurt	Organic plain yogurt with a little honey or fruit
Regular cereal	Ancient grains cereal (find a low sugar alternative preferably under 7g of added sugar per serving)
Flavored instant oatmeal	Organic plain oatmeal. You can add fruit, nuts, or seeds after it's cooked.
Fruit juices	Organic vegetable/fruit juice low in sugar (aim for less than 8g of sugar per serving)
Bottled sweetened iced tea	Use tea bags to prepare your tea and then refrigerate. Add a little honey if you need to sweeten.
Coffee or other caffeinated beverages	Green tea
Soda	Fruit infused water/carbonated water/Kombucha

Part Four
FEEL AMAZING AND LIVE AMAZINGLY

The power to create your best life is in your hands. All you need to do is show up for yourself and step into your powerful self. I believe that the Radiant Energy program will give you a jumpstart to health, but you must be willing to change your mind about the role you play in your life. Inspirational speaker Wayne Dyer once said: "Change the way you look at things and the things you look at change." Incredible transformation is always available to you. Believe it, and you will see it. Dare to honor yourself with unconditional love, trust and acceptance, and witness the miracles that come with that.

You are creation, you are pure energy, you are love, you are kindness, you are an extraordinary manifestation of the universe, and you are health. Make up your mind, and change your world for the better.

Chapter Twelve
RADIANT MOMMY

Mommies, it is time to shine. No longer will you believe this cranky, tired version of yourself is the best you can do as a mom. How are you supposed to live your best life if you are lukewarm or miserable? You can't, so let's change that.

The Radiant Energy program will help you hit the reset button and reclaim your vitality and glow. I urge you to stop using the band aid fix on everything. You cannot force wellness. It is a process that requires your participation every day. You must commit to yourself in a holistic way if you want to feel whole again. Your vibrant, beautiful self is in the sum of all your parts. It is radical self-love and all the health and joy that come with it.

I know how hard you work every day to support your family's success. You are kind, smart, strong, and focused on the well-being of those you love. Now I want you to turn inward and observe all the magic you are. I want you to tap into the goddess within. I invite you to connect with her so you can see you are one – an almighty woman, capable and deserving of her best life.

I would like to share this brief meditation to cement the confidence and self-love that come with recognizing all the beauty and power within yourself.

Connecting to the Goddess Within

Sit comfortably or lie down in a quiet and comfortable place.

Take a deep breath in, let it out slowly to the count of four, and close your eyes on that exhale.

With each breath you take (breathe normally; do not force the breath) say the following on your exhale (either in your head or out loud):

"I am love."

"I am strength."

"I am tenacity."

"I am creation."

"I am health."

Every time you say/think a statement visualize the words any way that feels right for you. You can visualize them as light of any color shining bright inside your chest. You can feel them as a vibration. Or it can just be a feeling. There is no wrong way to experience these statements, and it might be different every time. That is ok. Allow yourself that space to grow, feel, or just be in this brief moment with yourself.

Repeat this cycle at least twice.

When you are done take one more deep breath, exhale to the count of four and open your eyes.

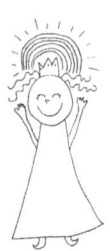

The Investment and the Payoff

Health is your most priceless commodity. The amount you are willing to invest in it determines how much you get. I am not talking about money, although at times it is warranted. How much time, dedication, and effort are you willing to put in in order to live in health?

You might feel like health is elusive, but it is not. Health is your natural state. If you connect and commit to yourself with love, kindness, respect, knowledge, and gratitude, you will experience health in its most powerful form. Your best life will not happen overnight. It will happen when you choose to constantly engage in the activities that nurture your body and soul. Give it a try. If you commit yourself to this program for three weeks, you will improve your mood, energy, skin, confidence, and zest for life.

I want you to feel connected to yourself and live the life you have always wanted now. I want you to welcome every day with a smile on your face and a heart filled with gratitude. I want you to feel like it is your 21st birthday, and you are oozing with confidence and health. I want you to feel inspired and radiant. So I want you to take the first step and jumpstart your journey to health. This is what this program is about. This incredible transformation is for you to make, and now you have the tools to do it. You might not be able to control what motherhood throws at you, but you can certainly take charge of your health. Health is your most valuable asset. Do not put it on the back burner.

You can heal and sustain health. An elevated mood, increased vitality, and radiant skin are all available to you. Take them. You can feel amazing and look amazing. Invest in your health. It always pays off.

The Ripple Effect for You and Your Children

When you treat yourself with kindness and respect your actions are aligned with radical self-love. This creates a cycle that flows with ease and all your actions will be motivated by that love. Caring for yourself will come naturally. Making good choices will not be hard work. It will be easy to eat nourishing foods because healing your body makes you feel good. It will be easier to go to bed early because you enjoy the vitality that comes with it. Making yourself a priority will not feel selfish because you know this vital act has a powerful ripple effect.

Now, I would like to ask you what kind of life you want for your children. If the words health, happiness, love, safety, respect, and self-love are somewhere in your answer, then you must ask yourself if these are things that you are allowing yourself to have. The way you live **your** life is the way you are teaching your kids to live theirs. When you live your best life, you are giving your children the best gift because you are teaching them how to live **their** best lives.

Living your most amazing life is rooted in choices made through self-love. Every day you are granted the gift of choice. Choose you. Your best life is waiting. Take it, Radiant Mommy, and spread this powerful ripple of health everywhere you go.

I am radiant
I am unlimited possibilities

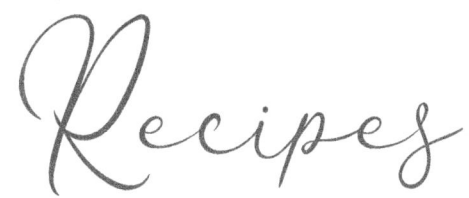

Breakfast Recipes

Power Up Omelet	102
Power Up Oatmeal	103
Avocado and Eggs	104
Breakfast Smoothie	105
Fruit and Yogurt Cup	106

Lunch Recipes

Omega-3 Power Salad	107
Zoodles and Chicken	108
Lentil Salad	109
Better Nachos	110
Roasted Carrot and Ginger Soup	111
Chicken and Kale Salad	112

Dinner Recipes

Roasted Cod and Sweet Potatoes	113
Seared Shrimp and Pumpkin Soup	114
Vegetarian Chili	116
Salmon with Green Goddess Quinoa Bowl	118
Vegetable and Tofu Stir Fry	120

Beverages and Broths for Radiant Skin

Magic Mineral Broth Recipe by Rebecca Katz	122
Turmeric and Orange Crush	124
Skin Detox Tea	126
Fruit Infused Water	127
Hydrating and Cleansing Juice	128
Bone Broth	129

Breakfast Recipes
POWER UP OMELET

INGREDIENTS:

- 2 eggs
- 1 cup of spinach
- ½ cup of sliced cremini mushrooms
- ¼ cup of chopped onion
- Organic butter
- Rosemary
- Himalayan salt and organic pepper

INSTRUCTIONS:

1. Heat butter in large skillet over medium-high heat.
2. Add mushrooms and onion; sauté for about 5 minutes.
3. Season with a little salt, pepper and rosemary.
4. Stir in baby spinach until wilted.
5. Transfer mushroom mixture to plate and wipe out skillet.
6. Mix eggs in a bowl.
7. Add 1 tbsp of butter to skillet.
8. Add the egg mixture and stir around the pan.
9. Cook about 2 minutes, until eggs are just slightly shiny on top.
10. Add mushroom and spinach mixture to one side of the omelet.
11. Lift up the edge of the omelet and fold it over the filling.
12. Slide omelet out of skillet and onto plate to serve.
13. You can top with organic parmesan cheese if you like.

POWER UP OATMEAL

INGREDIENTS:

- 1 cup of unflavored oatmeal
- Handful of blueberries and diced strawberries
- Handful of walnuts
- 1 tsp of chia seeds
- Cinnamon

INSTRUCTIONS:

1. Cook oatmeal according to instructions.
2. Once oatmeal is ready, serve in a bowl and add berries, nuts, chia seeds, and cinnamon to taste.

AVOCADO AND EGGS

INGREDIENTS:

- 2 eggs
- 1 avocado, halved and pitted
- 1 slice of turkey bacon, chopped up
- ½ a bell pepper, chopped
- Handful of diced chives

INSTRUCTIONS:

1. Place halved avocado pieces on plate.
2. Scramble eggs.
3. Place eggs on top of avocado pieces.
4. Top with bacon, pepper, and chives.
5. Add salt and pepper to taste.

BREAKFAST SMOOTHIE

INGREDIENTS:

- 1 banana
- 1 spoonful of peanut butter
- 1 cup of plain kefir or yogurt
- 1 tsp of cinnamon
- ½ spoonful of cocoa powder (no added sugar)
- ½ spoonful of raw honey
- Optional: high-quality whey or collagen protein

INSTRUCTIONS:

1. Add all ingredients to blender.
2. Blend.

FRUIT AND YOGURT CUP

INGREDIENTS:

- Fruits like berries, mangos, cherries, coconut, or kiwi (Use your favorites.)
- Plain whole milk yogurt or dairy-free alternative
- Granola, seeds (like sunflower, pumpkin, or chia) or ancient grain mix

INSTRUCTIONS:

1. Place layer of fruit mix in an 8-ounce mason jar.
2. Top with yogurt.
3. Add another layer of fruit.
4. Add another layer of yogurt.
5. Leave enough space on top to add granola/seeds.
6. Put the lid on without adding the granola/seeds. Refrigerate for at least 30 minutes or leave overnight.
7. When ready to eat, top with granola/seeds.

Lunch Recipes

OMEGA-3 POWER SALAD

INGREDIENTS:

- 1 lb. of canned, drained wild salmon
- 1 small cucumber, peeled and diced
- ¼ cup of diced onion
- 1 tbsp of olive oil
- Juice of half a lemon
- 1 tbsp of dill, parsley, or chives
- Two handfuls of spring salad mix

INSTRUCTIONS:

1. Combine all ingredients (except spring mix).
2. Place spring mix in a bowl and top with salmon mix.
3. Refrigerate leftovers for another meal.

ZOODLES AND CHICKEN

INGREDIENTS:

- Big handful of zucchini noodles (about one zucchini)
- 1 chopped garlic clove
- 1 spoonful of organic butter
- 1 organic chicken breast
- 1 tbsp of olive oil
- 1 small tomato, diced
- Grated organic parmesan to taste

INSTRUCTIONS:

1. Cook chicken breast to your liking, chop, and set aside.
2. In medium pan, melt butter, and sauté zucchini noodles and garlic for 3 to 5 minutes.
3. Remove from pan and serve.
4. Top with cooked chicken and diced tomato.
5. Add parmesan, salt, and pepper to taste.

LENTIL SALAD

INGREDIENTS:

- 1 cup of lentils
- 4 cups of water or broth
- 2 chopped carrots
- 2 chopped stalks of celery
- 1 cup of chopped bell peppers
- ¼ cup of olive oil
- Juice of one lemon
- Himalayan salt and organic pepper
- Pumpkin seeds

INSTRUCTIONS:

1. Cook lentils according to package instructions and drain.
2. Mix chopped vegetables with oil and lemon juice (you can also use a quality pre-made dressing like Bragg's Ginger and Sesame). Add lentils to mix. Salt and pepper to taste.
3. Refrigerate for 30 minutes or overnight.
4. When ready to eat, serve and top with pumpkin seeds.

BETTER NACHOS

INGREDIENTS:

- Multi-grain tortilla chips
- ½ an avocado in small cubes
- 1 small tomato, diced
- 1 celery stalk, chopped
- Handful of spring salad mix chopped
- Organic shredded cheese of your choice
- Spoonful of chia seeds

INSTRUCTIONS:

1. Place chips in a toaster-oven safe dish and layer with cheese. Place in toaster oven and heat till cheese melts.
2. Top with rest of ingredients. Consider adding a little sauerkraut for a probiotic power-up.

ROASTED CARROT AND GINGER SOUP

INGREDIENTS:

- 1 bag (one pound) of organic carrots
- 2-3 garlic cloves
- ½ an onion, chopped
- 2 cups of Magic Mineral Broth (can also use store bought vegetable broth)
- 1 tsp of grated ginger
- ½ cup of coconut milk
- Avocado oil
- Himalayan salt and organic pepper to taste

INSTRUCTIONS:

1. Peel and chop carrots.
2. Preheat oven to 350 degrees.
3. Place carrots, garlic, and onion on baking sheet. Top with avocado oil, and a little salt and pepper.
4. Roast for about 30 minutes or until carrots are soft.
5. Blend roasted vegetables and 1 cup of broth until smooth.
6. In large pot place vegetable blend, the rest of the broth, and coconut milk.
7. Simmer.
8. Add salt and pepper to taste.

CHICKEN AND KALE SALAD

INGREDIENTS:

BALSAMIC VINAIGRETTE DRESSING:
- Juice of 2 lemons
- 1 tbsp of Dijon mustard
- 2 tbsp of balsamic vinegar
- 2 cloves of garlic, fine chopped
- ¼ tsp of salt
- ¼ tsp of black pepper
- 1 tsp of honey
- ¼ cup of olive oil

CHICKEN SALAD:
- 1lb of organic chicken breast, cooked and cubed
- ½ a red onion, diced
- 2 cups of chopped broccoli
- ½ cup of sunflower seeds
- ½ cup of shredded carrots
- 1 cup of sliced cucumber
- 1 cup of diced tomato
- 1 cup of deseeded and diced yellow bell pepper
- 1 cup of brussels sprouts, rough chopped
- 5 cups of kale, cut and lightly mixed together with 1tbsp of olive oil

INSTRUCTIONS:

1. Mix all ingredients for dressing until well combined.
2. Mix all the ingredients for the salad adding the kale last.
3. Toss with dressing.

Dinner Recipes

ROASTED COD AND SWEET POTATOES

INGREDIENTS:

- Cod fillet
- Sweet potato
- Juice of half a lemon
- Himalayan salt and organic pepper to taste
- 2 garlic cloves, diced
- ½ tbsp of avocado oil
- ¼ tsp of paprika
- ¼ tsp of cinnamon

INSTRUCTIONS:

1. Preheat oven to 400 degrees.
2. Peel and dice sweet potato into even cubes and place in bowl.
3. Add avocado oil, paprika, cinnamon, 1 garlic clove (diced), and salt and pepper to taste.
4. Place seasoned sweet potatoes on baking sheet.
5. Roast potatoes for about 30-40 minutes, stirring every 10 minutes.

FOR COD:

1. Mix a spoonful of melted butter with lemon juice and 1 diced garlic clove.
2. Brush cod with butter mixture (add salt and pepper to taste) and place in oven about 20 minutes after you have placed the sweet potatoes.
3. Cook cod for about 15 minutes.
4. Remove cod and potatoes from oven when ready and serve along with your favorite salad.

SEARED SHRIMP AND PUMPKIN SOUP

INGREDIENTS:

SEARED SHRIMP:
- 1 lb. of fresh shrimp, peeled and deveined.
- 3 tsp of salt
- 3 tsp of garlic powder
- 1 tsp of onion powder
- 3 tsp of turmeric
- 1 tbsp of coconut oil

PUMPKIN SOUP:
- 3 tsp coconut oil
- 3 tsp fresh ginger, finely chopped
- 1 white onion, diced
- 5 cloves of garlic, chopped
- 3 sprigs of fresh thyme
- 2 sprigs of fresh oregano
- 2 tsp of salt
- 3 tsp of black pepper
- 2 tsp of raw honey
- 2 lbs. of pumpkin, peeled, deseeded, and diced
- 1 can of organic coconut cream (14oz)
- 2 cups of vegetable stock
- Garnish: Roasted pumpkin seeds

INSTRUCTIONS:

SEARED SHRIMP:
1. Marinate shrimp with spices for half an hour and then sear in a hot pan with the coconut oil.
2. Set aside.

PUMPKIN SOUP:
1. In a pot, over medium heat add the coconut oil. Then add the onion, garlic, ginger, thyme, and oregano, and cook with the lid on, stirring occasionally.
2. Add the pumpkin and stir the pot well. Cover with the lid and allow to cook for around five minutes.
3. Add the coconut milk and the vegetable broth and bring to a simmer.
4. Continue to cook until the pumpkin is tender.
5. Remove the pot from the heat and puree the soup.
6. Serve the soup with shrimp and pumpkin seeds.

VEGETARIAN CHILI

INGREDIENTS:

- 2 tbsp of avocado oil
- ½ yellow onion, diced
- 6 cloves of garlic chopped
- 2 tsp of cumin
- 1 tsp of paprika
- 1 tsp of Cayenne pepper
- 1 tbsp of chili powder
- 2 tsp dried oregano
- 1 tbsp black pepper
- 2 sprigs fresh thyme
- 6 oz can of tomato paste
- 5 Roma tomatoes, chopped
- Five cups of vegetable stock
- 1 tbsp cornstarch
- 2 roasted red bell peppers deseeded and skin peeled, diced
- 15 ounce can of black beans, drained
- 15 ounce can of chickpeas, drained
- 15 ounce can of kidney beans, drained

FINISH WITH:

- Fresh cilantro, chopped – to taste
- 1 jalapeño, fine diced
- Juice of 1 lime

INSTRUCTIONS:

1. Over a medium heat, cook onion and garlic until translucent. Add the cumin, paprika, cayenne, oregano, black pepper, thyme, and tomato paste and cook for three more minutes stirring continuously.
2. Add the tomatoes and let it cook for an additional 10 minutes or until tender.
3. Whisk one cup of vegetable stock with the cornstarch and set aside, pour the remaining four cups into the pot and allow to simmer for 15 minutes.
4. Whisk in the one cup of vegetable stock with the cornstarch; this will help to thicken the broth. Allow this to cook for another 5 minutes.
5. Add the roasted red bell peppers and then all of the beans and chickpeas and allow to cook for an additional 5 minutes.
6. Remove pot from heat and season to taste with fresh cilantro, jalapeno, and lime juice.

SALMON WITH GREEN GODDESS QUINOA BOWL

INGREDIENTS:

GREEN GODDESS DRESSING:
- 1 cup of organic mayonnaise/sour cream
- ¼ cup of buttermilk
- 3 tbsp of lime juice
- 3 cloves of garlic chopped
- ½ tsp of salt
- ½ cup chopped cilantro
- ¼ cup chopped basil
- ¼ cup chopped chives
- 3 chopped green onions
- 1 tsp of apple cider vinegar
- 1 tsp of honey

SALMON:
- 4 6oz salmon fillets
- 1 tsp of salt
- 2 tsp black pepper
- 4 cloves of chopped garlic
- Zest of 1 organic lemon
- 3 tbsp of olive oil

QUINOA BOWL:
- 3 tsp of olive oil
- 3 cloves of garlic, rough chopped
- 1 tsp of salt
- ½ cup of grape tomatoes, halved
- ¼ cup of brussels sprouts, sliced
- ¼ cup of yellow squash, diced
- 1 red bell pepper, sliced
- 3 cups of cooked quinoa

FINISH WITH:
- Fresh green onion, sliced

INSTRUCTIONS:

GREEN GODDESS DRESSING:
1. Mix all ingredients and set aside.

SALMON:
1. Marinate the salmon in the rest of the ingredients (listed under the salmon section of the ingredient list) for half an hour.
2. Set oven to 375 degrees.
3. Wrap each fillet in aluminum foil and place them on a tray.
4. Bake for 10-12 minutes and check fish. You can cook for a few more minutes if you prefer your fish well done.

QUINOA BOWL:
1. Heat the oil in a pan over medium heat. Add oil, salt, and garlic.
2. Once the garlic starts to sizzle, the oil is hot enough to add the tomatoes. Allow them to cook through until almost shriveled.
3. Add the brussels sprouts, squash, and red bell pepper and cook to al dente (still have a slight crunch).
4. Raise the heat to medium high and add the cooked quinoa.
5. Remove from heat once everything is completely heated through.
6. Serve with salmon fillets and add the green goddess dressing.

VEGETABLE AND TOFU STIR FRY

INGREDIENTS:

- 1 lb. of firm tofu
- 1 tbsp of coconut oil
- 3 tbsp of fresh ginger, chopped
- 3 cloves of garlic, chopped
- 1 shallot, fine diced
- 1 can of baby corn, halved (or use three ears of fresh corn kernels)
- 1 Thai chili (or 1 serrano chili), finely chopped
- 2 red bell peppers, chopped
- 2 carrots, chopped
- 1 cup Napa cabbage, thinly sliced
- 2 tbsp of low sodium soy sauce. You can replace soy sauce with Braggs Liquid Aminos.
- 3 tbsp hoisin sauce
- 1 tsp of honey

GARNISH:
- Lime juice
- Fresh cilantro
- Fresh basil

INSTRUCTIONS:

1. Wrap the tofu in paper towels to absorb as much moisture as possible and then set aside while prepping the other ingredients.
2. Remove the paper towel from the tofu and cut into 1 inch cubes.
3. When ready to cook heat the oil in a large pan and sear the cubed tofu. Once it has some color, add the ginger, garlic, and shallot and allow to cook for two minutes, stirring occasionally.
4. Add the remaining ingredients and cook until the sauce has thickened and the vegetables are cooked to al dente.
5. Finish with fresh lime juice, cilantro, and basil.
6. Serve with Basmati rice.

Beverages and Broths for Radiant Skin

MAGIC MINERAL BROTH RECIPE BY REBECCA KATZ

Reprinted with permission from The Cancer-Fighting Kitchen: Nourishing, Big-Flavor Recipes for Cancer Treatment and Recovery. Copyright © 2009 by Rebecca Katz with Mat Edelson, Ten Speed Press, a division of the Crown Publishing Group, Berkeley, CA. Makes 6 quarts

> The Magic Mineral Broth is a healing and nourishing elixir that can be used daily. Some of the benefits of this broth, rich in minerals like potassium and magnesium, are:
>
> - Soothes the nervous system
> - Boosts the immune system
> - Promotes gut health
> - Supports restful sleep
> - Nurturing for the body

INGREDIENTS:

- 6 unpeeled carrots, cut into thirds
- 2 unpeeled yellow onions, cut into chunks
- 1 leek, white and green parts, cut into thirds
- 1 bunch celery, including the heart, cut into thirds
- 4 unpeeled red potatoes, quartered
- 2 unpeeled Japanese or regular sweet potatoes, quartered
- 1 unpeeled garnet yam, quartered
- 5 unpeeled cloves of garlic, halved
- ½ bunch fresh flat-leaf parsley
- 1 (8-inch) strip of kombu (a mineral rich seaweed)
- 12 black peppercorns
- 4 whole all spice or juniper berries
- 2 bay leaves
- 8 quarts of cold, filtered water
- 1 tsp of sea salt

INSTRUCTIONS:

1. Rinse all of the vegetables. Put all ingredients in a stockpot. Fill the pot with water two inches below the rim, cover and bring to a boil.
2. Remove the lid, decrease the heat to low, and simmer uncovered for at least two hours. As the broth simmers, some of the water will evaporate; add more if the vegetables begin to peek out. Simmer until the full richness of the vegetables can be tasted. Strain the broth. Allow to cool. Then store in mason jars and refrigerate.

TURMERIC AND ORANGE CRUSH

INGREDIENTS:

- 2 cups of filtered water
- ½ to 1 tsp of turmeric powder
- Juice of ½ a freshly squeezed orange

INSTRUCTIONS:

1. Boil water.
2. Add turmeric powder and lower the heat.
3. Simmer for 10 minutes.
4. Strain the tea into a cup using a cheese cloth.
5. Add orange juice.

CINNAMON AND CHAMOMILE TEA

INGREDIENTS:

- 1 cinnamon stick
- 1 cup of water
- 1 chamomile tea bag
- For more servings add one cinnamon stick and chamomile bag per additional cup of water.

INSTRUCTIONS:

1. Heat water with cinnamon in it.
2. Pour hot water into cup with tea bag.
3. Add the cinnamon stick to the cup.
4. Sweetener is not required, but if you need a little more sweetness, add ½ tsp of raw honey.

SKIN DETOX TEA

INGREDIENTS:

- 2 sachets of peppermint tea
- 2 sachets of chamomile tea
- 2 cardamom pods
- 1 tsp of dried orange peel (optional)

INSTRUCTIONS:

1. Combine all in a jar and add boiling water. Allow to sit for two to three minutes. Then strain and serve.

FRUIT INFUSED WATER

INGREDIENTS:

- 1 organic cucumber, sliced
- 1 organic lemon, sliced
- 1 organic orange, sliced
- A handful of organic mint to taste

INSTRUCTIONS:

1. Put all ingredients in a 1 liter jar filled with filtered water and let sit overnight in the fridge.
2. You can create your own water infusions with watermelon, berries, ginger, or kiwi.

HYDRATING AND CLEANSING JUICE

INGREDIENTS:

- 3 large kale leaves or a cup of chopped kale
- 1 cucumber
- Small handful of parsley
- ½ lemon

INSTRUCTIONS:

1. Rinse all ingredients and put through juicer. Drink immediately.

BONE BROTH

There are many recipes for bone broth, and they are all pretty simple. You can do a quick search and find your favorite. Remember to always use bone sources that are organic. This is how I make it at home.

INGREDIENTS:

- Leftover bones from a whole organic chicken.

INSTRUCTIONS:

1. Place bones in crock pot and fill with filtered water.
2. Add one spoonful of vinegar and let sit for one hour (helps detach minerals from bones).
3. Cook on high heat for seven hours.
4. Remove bones from broth.
5. Sift broth into mason jars and refrigerate.

ABOUT / BIO

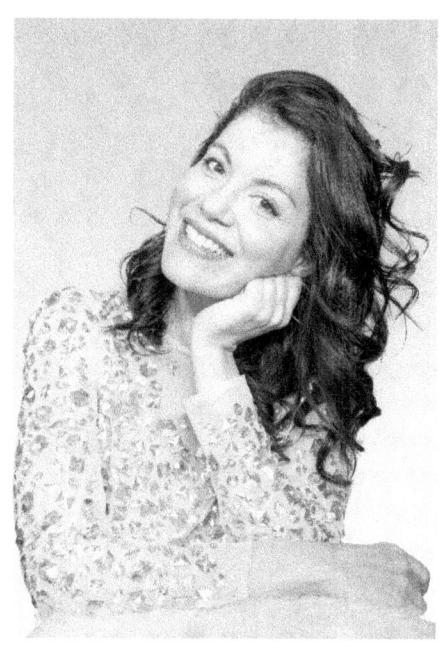

Ixiana Hernández Wilmot is the nutrition and lifestyle consultant behind the Radiant Mami brand, specializing in helping women create balance and health. She is a mom and a passionate advocate for women's health. Ixiana is fascinated by hormones and all things stress related, which is why her signature program, Radiant Energy, focuses on giving women a clear guide to stress reduction and supporting hormonal balance. She believes with information, action, trust, and lots of self-love, anything is possible. "All women are deserving and capable of living their best lives in health." is her motto. When she is not playing with her family, you will find her trying to change the world on her website www.radiantmami.com and on Instagram @radiant_mami and Radiant Mami on Facebook and YouTube. Ixiana has a health coaching degree and a Masters of Science in Holistic Nutrition.

RESOURCES

Environmental Working Group

The Environmental Working Group is a non-profit, non-partisan organization whose mission is to empower people to live healthier lives in a healthier environment. You can use their reports, databases, and mobile apps to make safer and more informed decisions about the products you buy. This website is full of resources to help you reduce your toxic load. I highly recommend it.

www.ewg.org
www.ewg.org/skindeep

Good Calculators

This website offers a collection of online calculators that can help you determine your status or needs for numerous health topics. Under the sports and health category, for example, you will find water intake and BMI calculators.

www.goodcalculators.com

Mindful

Mindful is a mission-driven non-profit dedicated to inspiring, guiding, and connecting people with the purpose of exploring mindfulness in order to enjoy better health, more caring relationships, and a compassionate society. On their website you can find free guided meditations and daily practices to cultivate mindfulness.

www.mindful.org

National Sleep Foundation

The National Sleep Foundation is a federal organization dedicated to improving health and well-being through sleep education and advocacy.
www.sleepfoundation.org

Self Nutrition Database

Nutrition Data is a good source to find detailed nutrition information plus unique analysis tools that tell you more about how foods affect your health. It also has a daily needs calculator to help you figure out the calories that you burn, your body mass index (BMI), and recommended daily values for key nutrients.
www.nutritiondata.self.com

Sugar Science

Sugar Science is the authoritative source for evidence-based, scientific information about sugar, and its impact on health.
www.sugascience.ucsf.edu

The World's Healthiest Foods

The George Mateljan Foundation is a not-for-profit foundation with a mission to help people eat and cook the healthiest way for optimal health. It is a great resource to find out about the nutrients found in foods, and how to prepare them.
www.whfoods.org/

World Health Organization

WHO is a worldwide organization dedicated to promoting health and safety and to serving the vulnerable. Their goals are to ensure that a billion more people have universal health coverage, to protect a billion more people from health emergencies, and to provide another billion people with better health and well-being.
www.who.int

Radiant Mami

The virtual headquarters for all Radiant Mami operations and information. This website shares my vision of motherhood in health, joy, and power by providing women with information, inspiration, and tools to take charge of their wellness journey. Together we can work to create nutrition and lifestyle habits that address stress and promote balance. For access to downloadable worksheets and print outs that enhance your book experience use the link https://www.radiantmami.com/book-extras or select book extras from the book drop down menu on www.radiantmami.com and enter the password: ICREATE.
www.radiantmami.com

GLOSSARY OF TERMS

ADDED SUGARS: Sugars that do not occur naturally in a food; they are added to enhance flavor.

ADDITIVES: A substance added to food in order to enhance or preserve it.

ADRENAL GLANDS: Hormone secreting glands located at the top of the kidneys.

ADRENALINE: A hormone secreted by the adrenal glands known as epinephrine. Its main function is to prepare the body for fight or flight. It increases blood circulation, breathing rate, and metabolism of carbohydrates.

ADRENOCORTICOTROPIC HORMONE (ACTH): A polypeptide tropic hormone produced in the pituitary gland. Its main function is to stimulate cortisol production.

AGAVE SYRUP: Sweetener made from the agave plant. Contrary to popular belief, it is not a healthier alternative to other sugars. It has a low glycemic load, but its high fructose content can be detrimental to the liver.

ANTI-INFLAMMATORY DIET: A diet based on foods that lower inflammation. It replaces sugary and refined foods with whole nutrient-rich foods. Antioxidants are a big component of the anti-inflammatory diet.

ANTI-NUTRIENTS: Natural or synthetic substances found in foods that can block the absorption of nutrients in the body.

ANTIOXIDANTS: Substances that inhibit oxidation.

ASTHMA: Chronic disease that affects the breathing pathways.

AUTOIMMUNE DISEASE: Condition that causes your immune system to malfunction and attack your own body and healthy cells.

AUTONOMIC NERVOUS SYSTEM: Part of the nervous system that regulates the functions of our internal organs without conscious effort. It has two main divisions: the sympathetic and parasympathetic.

CALORIE: A unit of heat used to measure the amount of energy released by a food.

CARBOHYDRATES: The body's main source of energy. Sugars, starches and fibers found in fruits, vegetables, grains, and dairy are carbohydrates.

CARDIAC: Related to the heart.

CATECHOLAMINES: Hormones synthesized in the adrenal glands. They include dopamine, epinephrine (adrenaline), and norepinephrine. If synthesized in the nervous system, they are considered neurotransmitters.

CENTRAL NERVOUS SYSTEM: Part of the nervous system composed of the brain and spinal cord. It plays a role in most body functions.

CHEMICAL: Process involving a reaction between multiple substances. Chemicals are the substances used or produced by a chemical process.

CHRONIC INFLAMMATION: Prolonged response by the immune system that causes a slow or long term inflammation.

CHRONIC STRESS: Prolonged body response to a stressor that involves the constant release of cortisol.

CIRCADIAN DISRUPTION: Disturbance on a molecular level that changes our body's circadian clock.

CIRCADIAN RHYTHM: The 24-hour cycle that regulates all physiological processes, including the sleep-wake cycle.

COGNITIVE: Relating to the mental process linked to thinking.

CORTICOTROPIN-RELEASE HORMONE (CRH): Peptide hormone secreted by the hypothalamus in response to stress. Its main function is to stimulate the secretion of ACTH.

CORTISOL: Glucocorticoid synthesized by the adrenal glands, also known as the "stress hormone." Most cells in the body have cortisol receptors, so cortisol affects many different bodily functions. Blood sugar levels, metabolism, memory formation, inflammation, water balance, and blood pressure are all influenced by cortisol.

DAMAGED FATS: Oxidized fats that contain free radicals and cause inflammation in the body. Fried foods and oils heated at high temperatures contain damaged fats.

DESENSITIZE: To make something less sensitive.

DETOXIFICATION PATHWAYS: Physiological routes for detoxification. The liver and kidneys are the main organs of detoxification in the body.

DHEA: Dehydroepiandrosterone is a hormone produced in the adrenal glands. Its main function is to assist in the production of sex hormones like testosterone and estrogen.

DYSFUNCTION: Abnormal or impaired function of an organ or system in the body.

ELECTRICAL BALANCE: Balance within electrolyte function.

ELECTROLYTES: Chemicals that conduct electricity in the body fluids. They regulate nerve and muscle function, keep the body hydrated, maintain blood acidity and pressure balance, and help in tissue repair.

ENTERIC NERVOUS SYSTEM: Part of the autonomic nervous system, it is composed of neurons all along the intestinal lining that control the gastrointestinal track.

FIBER: A carbohydrate that cannot be digested. It helps eliminate waste and maintain balance in the body. Fiber can be catalogued as soluble and insoluble.

FIGHT OR FLIGHT RESPONSE: Physiological reaction to stress that activates the sympathetic nervous system in order to prepare the body for survival.

FREE RADICALS: Unstable molecular species containing an unpaired electron.

GENETICALLY MODIFIED ORGANISM (GMO): Organisms that have been artificially manipulated by combining genes from different organisms. The top concerns about negative effects of GM foods on health are the transfer of antibiotic resistance, toxicity, and allergens.

GLUCOCORTICOIDS: A class of steroid hormone.

GLUCOSE: A simple sugar.

GLUTEN: A protein found in wheat. It acts as a binder and extending agent and is often used as an additive in processed foods to improve texture, flavor, and moisture retention. It can be difficult for the body to process gluten, and as a result, it can cause inflammation and distress in the digestive track.

GLYCEMIC DISTURBANCES: Conditions caused by problems with sugar regulation in the body. Hypoglycemia (very low sugar levels) and hyperglycemia (very high blood sugar levels) are both glycemic disturbances.

GLYCEMIC IMPACT: The weight of glucose that causes a glycemic response equivalent to that induced by a given amount of food. It refers to how a serving of food affects sugar levels in the blood.

GLYCEMIC LOAD: A measurement of the impact of a given amount of food on blood sugar levels after consumption. It takes into account the quality and quantity of the carbohydrate. Foods with a low glycemic load allow for a steadier release of sugar in the blood. Foods with a high glycemic load increase sugar levels rapidly, causing a spike in blood sugar.

HORMONES: A chemical substance produced by living cells that controls and regulates the activity of certain cells or organs. They are your body's chemical messengers.

HYPOTHALAMIC PITUITARY ADRENAL (HPA) AXIS: Neuroendocrine unit made up of the hypothalamus, the pituitary gland, and the adrenal glands. It is one of the main pathways for the stress response.

HYPOTHALAMUS: Region of the brain responsible for many important functions like hormone synthesis, regulation of temperature, circadian rhythm, appetite, and emotional responses. It is located at the base of the brain, next to the pituitary gland.

INFLAMMATORY SIGNALS: Cascade of chemical signals that stimulate the activation of the inflammatory response.

INSULIN: Hormone made in the pancreas that regulates glucose levels and utilization.

INSULIN RESISTANCE: Impaired ability of cells to respond to insulin that causes high blood sugar levels.

INSULIN SENSITIVITY: How sensitive the cells are to insulin.

INTESTINAL PERMEABILITY: Refers to the ability of substances to pass from the intestinal track to the body.

INVISIBLE LABOR: Physical and emotional labor involved in raising a family and taking care of the home.

IONS: An atom or molecule that has a net electrical charge.

KOMBUCHA: Beverage that results from the fermentation of tea using yeast and bacteria.

LIPIDS: Group of organic compounds that are greasy to the touch, insoluble in water, and soluble in alcohol and ether. Fats and oils are lipids.

LYMPHATIC SYSTEM: Part of the vascular system that transports lymph throughout the body. The main functions of this system are the removal of toxins, the absorbing and transporting of fatty acids, and the production and transport of immune cells.

MACULAR: Relating to the eye.

METABOLIC DISORDER: Disruption in metabolic function caused by abnormal chemical reactions. The most common metabolic disorder is diabetes.

METABOLIC SYNDROME: An array of conditions that increase the risk of heart disease, type 2 diabetes, fatty liver, and some cancers. Insulin resistance, central obesity, hypertension, and elevated levels of cholesterol or fats are the components of metabolic syndrome.

METABOLIC TOXINS: Waste substances from the body's metabolic processes.

METABOLISM: The whole range of biochemical processes that occur within a living organism.

MINDFULNESS: The practice of paying attention to the present moment.

MINDFULNESS BASED STRESS REDUCTION: Eight-week program that offers evidence-based intensive mindfulness training to help individuals address stress, anxiety, depression, and pain.

MINDSET: A person's point of view or life philosophy.

MINERALS: Inorganic nutrients that are essential for growth and health.

NEGATIVE FEEDBACK: Reaction that causes a reduced or decreased function.

NEURONS: Nerve cells that transmit information throughout the body.

NEUROTRANSMITTERS: Chemical messengers that are released at the end of a nerve fiber due to stimuli. They transmit messages between neurons or to muscles.

NUTRIENT: Substance that provides nourishment.

NUTRIENT DEPLETING FOODS: Foods that use up nutrients in the body instead of providing nutrients to the body.

OMEGA-3 FATS: A class of essential fatty acids that you must get from your diet. The most important are ALA (found in vegetable oils like flaxseed, coconut or avocado), DHA and EPA (found in seafood like fatty fish and algae).

ORGANIC FOODS: Grown without the use of pesticides, synthetic fertilizers, sewage sludge, genetically modified organisms, or ionizing radiation. Organic meat, poultry, eggs, and dairy products come from animals that are given no antibiotics or growth hormones.

OXIDATIVE STRESS (OS): An imbalance between the production of free radicals and the body's capability to neutralize them.

OXYTOCIN: Hormone and neurotransmitter synthesized in the hypothalamus and secreted by the pituitary gland. It plays a role in the female reproductive system and it can have an effect on social behaviors.

PHTHALATES: Chemicals used mainly as solvents and to make plastic flexible, transparent and durable. Aside from plastics, phthalates can be found in cosmetics, household cleaners, and personal care products. Some phthalates have been found to be hormone disruptors and toxic to humans.

PHYTONUTRIENTS: Plant-based compounds known to have antioxidant and anti-inflammatory benefits.

PITUITARY GLAND: Small gland found at the base of the brain. Also known as the master gland, the pituitary gland controls the function of most other endocrine glands.

PRESERVATIVES: Substance used in foods, cosmetics, pharmaceuticals, and other materials to prevent decay or unwanted chemical changes.

PROCESSED FOODS: Foods that have been changed from its original form by chemical or mechanical procedures.

PROTEIN: Essential macronutrient mainly composed of amino acids.

REFINED FOODS: Highly processed foods that have been stripped of fiber and their original nutrient content.

RUMINATION: Obsessive thinking about the causes and consequences of one's distress.

STRESS SIGNALS: Behaviors, feelings, thoughts, and physiological manifestations that signal a stress reaction.

STRESSOR: Emotional or physical stimuli that causes a stress reaction.

SUCROSE: Molecule made up of glucose and fructose that naturally occurs in plants.

TOXINS: Poisonous substances formed internally by cells or tissue (endotoxin), by an external source (exotoxin) or by a combination of both.

TRANSITION FOODS: Foods that can be used to substitute for harmful foods during the process of making a change to a healthier diet.

TRYPTOPHAN: Essential amino acid used in the biosynthesis of proteins.

VISCERAL ADIPOSITY: Excess fat in the abdominal area.

VITALITY: Exuberant energy and strength. Meaningful and purposeful living.

ZEITGEBERS: Environmental cue that regulates the body's circadian rhythms.

END NOTES

1. Salleh M. R. (2008). Life event, stress and illness. *The Malaysian journal of medical sciences: MJMS,15*(4), 9–18.
2. Ciciolla, L. & Luthar, S.S.(2019).Invisible Household Labor and Ramifications for Adjustment: Mothers as Captains of Households. *Sex Roles*, 0360 (0025), 1-20 https://doi.org/10.1007/s11199-018-1001
3. Joseph, D. N., & Whirledge, S. (2017). Stress and the HPA Axis: Balancing Homeostasis and Fertility. *International journal of molecular sciences, 18*(10), 2224. doi:10.3390/ijms18102224
4. Veldhuis, J. D., Sharma, A., & Roelfsema, F. (2013). Age-dependent and gender-dependent regulation of hypothalamic-adrenocorticotropic-adrenal axis. *Endocrinology and metabolism clinics of North America, 42*(2), 201–225. doi:10.1016/j.ecl.2013.02.002
5. National Women's Law Center (2017). A Snapshot of Working Mothers. Retrieved from: https://nwlc.org/wp-content/uploads/2017/04/A-Snapshot-of-Working-Mothers.pdf
6. Escalante Alison (2019) Mothers are drowning in stress; new research suggests saving U.S. mothers should be a national priority. *Psychology Today.* Retrieved from: https://www.psychologytoday.com/us/blog/shouldstorm/201903/mothers-are-drowning-in-stress
7. Everyday Health (2017) Everyday Health Launches A "Special Report on Women's Wellness" Shedding Necessary Light On What Defines Her Well Being In Today's Uncertain Climate. Retrieved from:https://www.prnewswire.com/news-releases/everyday-health-launches-a-special-report-on-womens-wellness-shedding-necessary-light-on-what-defines-her-well-being-in-todays-uncertain-climate-300571982.html
8. Henderson, A., Harmon, S. & Newman, H.(2016) The Price Mothers Pay, Even When They Are Not Buying It: Mental Health Consequences of Idealized Motherhood. *Sex Roles* 74: 512. https://doi.org/10.1007/s11199-015-0534-5

9. American Psychological Association (2018) Stress in America, Generation Z. Retrieved from: https://www.apa.org/news/press/releases/stress/2018/stress-gen-z.pdf
10. Barroso, N. E., Mendez, L., Graziano, P. A., & Bagner, D. M. (2018). Parenting Stress through the Lens of Different Clinical Groups: a Systematic Review & Meta-Analysis. *Journal of abnormal child psychology, 46*(3), 449–461. doi:10.1007/s10802-017-0313-6
11. Guilliams Tomas G. (2018) The Role of Stress and the HPA Axis in Chronic Disease Management. The Point Institute, Stevens Point, WI
12. Hubert, S., & Aujoulat, I. (2018). Parental Burnout: When Exhausted Mothers Open Up. *Frontiers in psychology, 9*, 1021. doi:10.3389/fpsyg.2018.01021
13. Kumar, A., Rinwa, P., Kaur, G., & Machawal, L. (2013). Stress: Neurobiology, consequences, and management. *Journal of pharmacy & bioallied sciences, 5*(2), 91–97. doi:10.4103/0975-7406.111818
14. Cheng, S.-T., Tsui, P. K., & Lam, J. H. M. (2015). Improving mental health in health care practitioners: Randomized controlled trial of a gratitude intervention. Journal of Consulting and Clinical Psychology, 83(1), 177-186. http://dx.doi.org/10.1037/a0037895
15. Stefan Salzmann, Frank Euteneur, Jana Strahler, Johannes A.C. Lafterton, Urs M. Nater & Winfried Rief. (2018) Optimizing expectations and distraction lead to lower cortisol levels after acute stress. Psychoneuroendocrinology. 88:144-152. doi: 10.1016/j.psyneuen.2017.12.011
16. Institute of Medicine (US) Committee on Sleep Medicine and Research; Colten HR, Altevogt BM, editors. Sleep Disorders and Sleep Deprivation: An Unmet Public Health Problem. Washington (DC): National Academies Press (US); 2006. 3, Extent and Health Consequences of Chronic Sleep Loss and Sleep Disorders. Available from: https://www.ncbi.nlm.nih.gov/books/NBK19961/
17. Serin Y, Acar Tek N: Effect of Circadian Rhythm on Metabolic Processes and the Regulation of Energy Balance. Ann Nutr Metab 2019;74:322-330. doi: 10.1159/000500071
18. Mohawk JA, Takahashi JS. Cell autonomy and synchrony of suprachiasmatic nucleus circadian oscillators. *Trends Neurosci* **34**: 349-358, 2011.

19. Schwartz W.J., Tavakoli-Nezhad M., Lambert C.M., Weaver D.R., de la Iglesia H.O. (2011)Distinct patterns of period gene expression in the suprachiasmatic nucleus underlie circadian clock photoentrainment by advances or delays. Proc. Natl Acad. Sci. U S A, 108, 17219–17224
20. Wehrens, S., Christou, S., Isherwood, C., Middleton, B., Gibbs, M. A., Archer, S. N., Skene, D. J., & Johnston, J. D. (2017). Meal Timing Regulates the Human Circadian System. Current biology : CB, 27(12), 1768–1775.e3. https://doi.org/10.1016/j.cub.2017.04.059
21. Kinsey, A. W., & Ormsbee, M. J. (2015). The health impact of nighttime eating: old and new perspectives. Nutrients, 7(4), 2648–2662. https://doi.org/10.3390/nu7042648
22. Potter, G. D., Skene, D. J., Arendt, J., Cade, J. E., Grant, P. J., & Hardie, L. J. (2016). Circadian Rhythm and Sleep Disruption: Causes, Metabolic Consequences, and Countermeasures. Endocrine reviews, 37(6), 584–608. https://doi.org/10.1210/er.2016-1083
23. Guilliams Tomas G. (2018) The Role of Stress and the HPA Axis in Chronic Disease Management. The Point Institute, Stevens Point, WI
24. Adam, T. C., Hasson, R. E., Ventura, E. E., Toledo-Corral, C., Le, K. A., Mahurkar, S., ... Goran, M. I., (2010). Cortisol is negatively associated with insulin sensitivity in overweight Latino youth. *The Journal of clinical endocrinology and metabolism, 95*(10), 4729–4735. doi:10.1210/jc.2010-0322
25. Rosmond, Roland. (2003). Stress induced disturbances of the HPA axis: A pathway to Type 2 diabetes?. Medical science monitor : international medical journal of experimental and clinical research. 9. RA35-9.
26. Guilliams Tomas G. (2018) The Role of Stress and the HPA Axis in Chronic Disease Management. The Point Institute, Stevens Point, WI p.81
27. Lindmark, S., Lönn, L., Wiklund, U., Tufvesson, M., Olsson, T. and Eriksson, J. W. (2005), Dysregulation of the Autonomic Nervous System Can Be a Link between Visceral Adiposity and Insulin Resistance. Obesity Research, 13: 717-728. doi:10.1038/oby.2005.81
28. Robert M. Sapolsky, L. Michael Romero, Allan U. Munck, How Do Glucocorticoids Influence Stress Responses? Integrating Permissive, Suppressive, Stimulatory, and Preparative Actions, *Endocrine Reviews*, Volume 21, Issue 1, 1 February 2000, Pages 55–89, https://doi.org/10.1210/edrv.21.1.0389

29. Guilliams Tomas G. (2018) The Role of Stress and the HPA Axis in Chronic Disease Management. The Point Institute, Stevens Point, WI
30. Roma Pahwa, Ishwarlal Jialal (2018). Chronic Inflammation. Stat Pearls. Retrieved from: https://www.ncbi.nlm.nih.gov/books/NBK493173/
31. Lobo, V., Patil, A., Phatak, A., & Chandra, N. (2010). Free radicals, antioxidants, and functional foods: Impact on human health. *Pharmacognosy reviews, 4*(8), 118–126. doi:10.4103/0973-7847.70902
32. Liguori, I., Russo, G., Curcio, F., Bulli, G., Aran, L., Della-Morte, D., ... Abete, P., (2018). Oxidative stress, aging, and diseases. *Clinical interventions in aging, 13*, 757–772. doi:10.2147/CIA.S158513
33. Sullivan Kelly (2017). Sleep Duration and Feeling Rested are Differentially Associated with Having Children Among Men and Women. *American Academy of Neurology.* Retrieved from: https://www.aan.com/PressRoom/Home/PressRelease/1527
34. National Sleep Foundation Recommends New Sleep Times. (2015) National Sleep Foundation. Retrieved from: https://www.sleepfoundation.org/press-release/national-sleep-foundation-recommends-new-sleep-times
35. Grandjean P., (1992). Individual susceptibility to toxicity. *Toxicology Letters.* 64 & 65, 43-5. https://doi.org/10.1016/0378-4274(92)90171-F
36. Cline John C. (2015) Nutrition, Detox, and Clinical Practice. *Alternative Therapies.* Vol 21, 3 Retrieved from: https://pdfs.semanticscholar.org/033c/18c84b636747c971adcec6811902350c760f.pdf
37. Nutrition Facts (n.d.). Standard American Diet. Retrieved on April 2019 from https://nutritionfacts.org/topics/standard-american-diet/
38. Hodges, R. E., & Minich, D. M. (2015). Modulation of Metabolic Detoxification Pathways Using Foods and Food-Derived Components: A Scientific Review with Clinical Application.*Journal of nutrition and metabolism,2015*, 760689. doi:10.1155/2015/760689
39. Krohn Jacqueline & Taylor Frances (2000). Water and Air. *Natural Detoxification.* (pp.143) Vancouver, BC Hartley & Marks Publishers Inc.
40. Skin Store, (2017). How Much Is Your Face Worth? Our Survey Results Revealed! Retrieved from: https://www.skinstore.com/blog/skincare/womens-face-worth-survey-2017/
41. Zota, A. R., & Shamasunder, B. (2017). The environmental injustice of beauty: framing chemical exposures from beauty products as a health disparities concern. *American journal of obstetrics and gynecology, 217*(4), 418.e1–418.e6. doi:10.1016/j.ajog.2017.07.020

42. Stephens, M. A., & Wand, G. (2012). Stress and the HPA axis: role of glucocorticoids in alcohol dependence. *Alcohol research : current reviews, 34*(4), 468–483.
43. Watkins E. R. (2008). Constructive and unconstructive repetitive thought. *Psychological bulletin,*134(2), 163–206. doi:10.1037/0033-2909.134.2.163
44. American Psychological Association. (2019). *Stress effects on the body.* http://www.apa.org/helpcenter/stress-body
45. Crum, A. J., Salovey, P., & Achor, S. (2013). Rethinking stress: The role of mindsets in determining the stress response. *Journal of Personality and Social Psychology,* 104(4), 716-733. http://dx.doi.org/10.1037/a0031201
46. Burford, N. G., Webster, N. A., & Cruz-Topete, D. (2017). Hypothalamic-Pituitary-Adrenal Axis Modulation of Glucocorticoids in the Cardiovascular System. *International journal of molecular sciences,18*(10), 2150. doi:10.3390/ijms18102150
47. Omega-3 and omega-6 fatty acid levels in depressive and anxiety disorders. Carisha S. Thesing, Mariska Bot, Yuri Milaneschi, Erik J. Giltay, Brenda W. J. H. Penninx. Psychoneuroendocrinology.2017 Oct 6;87: 53–62.Published online 2017 Oct 6.doi:10.1016/j.psyneuen.2017.10.005
48. Yanek, L. R., Kral, B. G., Moy, T. F., Vaidya, D., Lazo, M., Becker, L. C., & Becker, D. M. (2013). Effect of positive well-being on the incidence of symptomatic coronary artery disease. *The American journal of cardiology, 112*(8), 1120–1125. doi:10.1016/j.amjcard,2013.05.055
49. Kang, D.-H., Davidson, R. J., Coe, C. L., Wheeler, R. E., Tomarken, A. J., & Ershler, W. B. (1991). Frontal brain asymmetry and immune function. Behavioral Neuroscience, 105(6), 860-869. http://dx.doi.org/10.1037/0735-7044.105.6.860
50. Furness J.B., Callaghan B.P., Rivera L.R., Cho HJ. (2014) The Enteric Nervous System and Gastrointestinal Innervation: Integrated Local and Central Control. In: Lyte M., Cryan J. (eds) Microbial Endocrinology: The Microbiota-Gut-Brain Axis in Health and Disease. Advances in Experimental Medicine and Biology, vol 817. Springer, New York, NY
51. Harvard Health Publishing (2019) Stress and the sensitive gut. Retrieved from: https://www.health.harvard.edu/newsletter_article/stress-and-the-sensitive-gut
52. Du J, Huang J, An Y, Xu W (2018) The relationship between stress and negative emotion: The Mediating role of rumination. Clin Res Trials 4: doi: 10.15761/CRT.1000208

53. Seaward Brian Luke (2014) Reframing, creating a positive mindset. *Essentials of Managing Stress.* Jones & Bartlett Learning, Burlington, MA. pp.112
54. Emmons Robert A., Stern Robin (2013). GratitudeasaPsychotherapeutic Intervention. *JOURNAL OF CLINICAL PSYCHOLOGY: IN SESSION*, Vol. 69(8), 846–855
55. Vago David R., Silberweig David A. (2012). Self-awareness, self-regulation, and self-transcendence (S-ART): a framework for understanding the neurobiological mechanisms of mindfulness. *Functional Neuroimaging Laboratory, Department of Psychiatry, Brigham and Women's Hospital, Boston, MA, USA.* https://doi.org/10.3389/fnhum.2012.00296
56. National Center for Complimentary and Integrative Health (2019). Meditation: in depth. Retrieved from: https://nccih.nih.gov/health/meditation/overview.htm#hed3
57. Post Stephen G. (2005). Altruism, Happiness, and Health: It's Good to Be Good. International Journal of Behavioral Medicine.Vol. 12, No. 2, 66–77
58. Takahashi Toku, Babygirija Reji Reji, & Ludwig Kirk (2015). Anti-stress effect of hypothalamic oxytocin -Importance of somatosensory stimulation and social buffering. *International Journal of Neurology Research.* Vol 1, No 3. http://ghrnet.org/index.php/ijnr/article/view/1090
59. Post Stephen G. (2005). Altruism, Happiness, and Health: It's Good to Be Good. International *Journal of Behavioral Medicine.*Vol. 12, No. 2, 66–77
60. Cascio, C. N., O'Donnell, M. B., Tinney, F. J., Lieberman, M. D., Taylor, S. E., Strecher, V. J., & Falk, E. B. (2016). Self-affirmation activates brain systems associated with self-related processing and reward and is reinforced by future orientation. *Social cognitive and affective neuroscience,11*(4), 621–629. doi:10.1093/scan/nsv136
61. Schunk Dale H. (2001). Self-Regulation Through Goal Setting. *ERIC Digests.* Retrieved from: https://www.counseling.org/resources/library/eric%20digests/2001-08.pdf
62. Dominican University (2015). Study focuses on strategies for achieving goals, resolutions. Retrieved from: https://www.dominican.edu/dominicannews/study-highlights-strategies-for-achieving-goals
63. Keshavarz Afshar, M., Behboodi Moghadam, Z., Taghizadeh, Z., Bekhradi, R., Montazeri, A., & Mokhtari, P. (2015). Lavender fragrance essential oil and the quality of sleep in postpartum women. *Iranian Red Crescent medical journal, 17*(4), e25880. doi:10.5812/ircmj.17(4)2015.25880

64. Chien, L. W., Cheng, S. L., & Liu, C. F. (2012). The effect of lavender aromatherapy on autonomic nervous system in midlife women with insomnia. *Evidence-based complementary and alternative medicine : eCAM, 2012*, 740813. doi:10.1155/2012/740813
65. Jodi A. Mindell, Lorena S. Telofski, Benjamin Wiegand, Ellen S. Kurtz, A Nightly Bedtime Routine: Impact on Sleep in Young Children and Maternal Mood, *Sleep*, Volume 32, Issue 5, May 2009, Pages 599–606, https://doi.org/10.1093/sleep/32.5.599
66. Ruddick -Collins L.C., Johnston J.D., & Johnston A.M. (2018) The Big Breakfast Study: Chrono-nutrition influence on energy expenditure and body weight. *Nutrition Bulletin*. 43(2):174-183. doi: 10 1111/nbu.12323
67. Crosby, P., Hamnett, R., Putker, M., Hoyle, N. P., Reed, M., Karam, C. J., O'Neill, J. S. (2019). Insulin/IGF-1 Drives PERIOD Synthesis to Entrain Circadian Rhythms with Feeding Time. *Cell, 177*(4), 896–909.e20. doi:10.1016/j.cell.2019.02.017
68. Daniela Jakubowicz, Julio Wainstein, Zohar Landau, Itamar Raz, Bo Ahren, Nava Chapnik, Tali Ganz, Miriam Menaged, Maayan Barnea, Yosefa Bar-Dayan, Oren Froy (2017). Influences of Breakfast on Clock Gene Expression and Postprandial Glycemia in Healthy Individuals and Individuals With Diabetes: A Randomized Clinical Trial. *Diabetes Care*, 40 (11) 1573-1579; **DOI**: 10.2337/dc16-2753
69. Potter, G. D., Skene, D. J., Arendt, J., Cade, J. E , Grant, P. J., & Hardie, L. J. (2016). Circadian Rhythm and Sleep Disruption: Causes, Metabolic Consequences, and Countermeasures.*Endocrine reviews,37*(6), 584–608. doi:10.1210/er.2016-1083
70. Karolina Janků, Michal Šmotek, Eva Fárková & Jana Kopřivová (2019) Block the light and sleep well: Evening blue light filtration as a part of cognitive behavioral therapy for insomnia, Chronobiology International, DOI: 10.1080/07420528.2019.1692859
71. Shechter, A., Kim, E. W., St-Onge, M. P., & Westwood, A. J. (2018). Blocking nocturnal blue light for insomnia: A randomized controlled trial. *Journal of psychiatric research, 96*, 196–202. doi:10.1016/j.jpsychires.2017.10.015
72. Krohn Jacqueline & Taylor Frances (2000). Phases of Detoxification. *Natural Detoxification*. (pp.33-36) Vancouver, BC Hartley & Marks Publishers Inc.
73. Rakel David (2012). Detoxification. *Integrative Medicine*. (pp.922-924) Philadelphia, PA Elsevier Saunders.

74. Benefits of Exercise (2019). NIH U.S. National Library of Medicine. Retrieved from: https://medlineplus.gov/benefitsofexercise.html
75. Wingfield, H.L., Smith-Ryan, A.E., Melvin, M.N., Roelofs, E.J., Trexler, E.T., Hackney, A.C., Weaver, M.A., & Ryan, E.D. (2015). The acute effect of exercise modality and nutrition manipulations on post-exercise resting energy expenditure and respiratory exchange ratio in women: a randomized trial. *Sports Medicine – Open*.
76. Nutrients and bioactives in green leafy vegetables and cognitive decline. Martha Clare Morris, Yamin Wang, Lisa L. Barnes, David A. Bennett, Bess Dawson-Hughes, Sarah L. Booth. Neurology Jan 2018, 90 (3) e214-e222; DOI:10.1212/WNL.0000000000004815
77. Beiser, M. (2016). Longitudinal Research to Promote Effective Refugee Resettlement. *Transcultural Psychiatry*, 5, 56–71. https://doi.org/10.1177/1363461506061757
78. Yan Lin (2016) Dark Green Leafy Vegetables. Agricultural Research Service. Retrieved from: https://www.ars.usda.gov/plains-area/gfnd/gfhnrc/docs/news-2013/dark-green-leafy-vegetables/
79. Jones, D. L., Cross, P., Withers, P. J., DeLuca, T. H., Robinson, D. A., Quilliam, R. S., Harris, I. M., Chadwick, D. R. and Edwards-Jones, G. (2013), REVIEW: Nutrient stripping: the global disparity between food security and soil nutrient stocks. J Appl Ecol, 50: 851-862. doi:10.1111/1365-2664.12089
80. Šimoliūnas, E., Rinkūnaitė, I., Bukelskienė, Ž., & Bukelskienė, V. (2019). Bioavailability of Different Vitamin D Oral Supplements in Laboratory Animal Model. *Medicina (Kaunas, Lithuania), 55*(6), 265. doi:10.3390/medicina55060265
81. Jess A Gwin, Heather J Leidy, Breakfast Consumption Augments Appetite, Eating Behavior, and Exploratory Markers of Sleep Quality Compared with Skipping Breakfast in Healthy Young Adults, *Current Developments in Nutrition*, Volume 2, Issue 11, November 2018, nzy074, https://doi.org/10.1093/cdn/nzy074
82. Hawley Aubree (2018) Protein, Its What's for Breakfast. *American Society for Nutrition*. Retrieved from: https://nutrition.org/protein-its-whats-for-breakfast/

INDEX

A

Accountability 51
Added Sugars 34, 35, 37, 66, 67, 68, 69, 70, 77, 93, 137
Additives 34, 67, 82, 137
Adrenal Glands 19, 27, 137, 138, 139, 141
Adrenaline 18, 29, 137, 138
Adrenocorticotropic Hormone (ACTH) 20, 137
Agave 68, 70, 137
Anti-Inflammatory Diet 35, 137
Anti-Nutrients 67, 137
Antioxidants 29, 33, 35, 37, 62, 137, 138
Autonomic Nervous System 37, 58, 138, 140

B

Balance 12, 17, 18, 25, 27, 31, 32, 33, 35, 36, 37, 40, 47, 53, 54, 56, 61, 63, 65, 71, 75, 78, 131, 135, 139, 140

C

Carbohydrate 140, 141
Celiac Disease 82
Central Nervous System 46, 138
Chemicals 18, 22, 35, 67, 71, 138, 139, 144
Chronic Inflammation 28, 29, 138
Chronic Stress 15, 20, 25, 29, 49, 53, 138
Circadian Disruption 25, 26, 138
Circadian Rhythm 26, 27, 32, 33, 57, 63, 75, 139, 141
Cognitive Function 12, 20, 26, 29, 79
Corticotropin-Release Hormone (CRH) 20, 139
Cortisol 18, 20, 26, 27, 28, 29, 137, 138, 139

D

Detoxification 20, 29, 32, 33, 34, 35, 53, 54, 65, 70, 71, 72, 73, 74, 77, 78, 90, 139
    Detoxification Pathways 65, 139
DHEA 20, 139
Diabetes 26, 28, 67, 142

E

Enteric Nervous System 46, 140

F

Fatigue 16, 20, 25, 26, 28, 29, 54, 57, 65, 74, 82, 86
Fats 29, 34, 35, 37, 66, 67, 77, 78, 82, 86, 90, 93, 139, 142, 143
    Damaged Fats 37, 66, 67, 77, 90, 93, 139
    Trans Fats 34, 66
Fiber 34, 35, 62, 86, 90, 140, 143, 144
Fight or Flight Response 12, 140
Food Sensitivities 65, 82, 83
Free Radicals 29, 139, 140, 143

G

Glucose 26, 27, 68, 140, 141, 145
Glycemic 37, 137, 140, 141
    Glycemic Disturbances 140
    Glycemic Impact 37, 141
    Glycemic Load 137, 141
Goals 49, 51, 55, 56, 59, 85, 86, 135
Gratitude 26, 36, 47, 50, 63, 64, 84, 98

H

Heart Disease 28, 67, 142
Hormones 12, 19, 20, 29, 33, 49, 53, 61, 66, 70, 86, 131, 138, 139, 141, 143
    Hormonal Pathways 26
Hypothalamic Pituitary Adrenal (HPA) Axis 12, 18, 19, 20, 25, 27, 28, 29, 30, 32, 33, 36, 37, 47, 53, 65, 141
Hypothalamus 19, 20, 26, 139, 141, 144

I

Inflammation 15, 25, 26, 28, 29, 33, 35, 54, 65, 66, 73, 137, 138, 139, 140
    Inflammatory Signals 28, 29, 33, 141
Insulin 27, 28, 61, 86, 141, 142
    Insulin Resistance 28, 141, 142
    Insulin Sensitivity 27, 141
Intestinal Permeability 29, 141
Invisible Labor 17, 142

L

Lipids 29, 142
Lymphatic System 65, 72, 142

M

Macular 79, 142
Metabolic 18, 28, 29, 37, 142
    Metabolic Disorder 29, 142
    Metabolic Syndrome 28, 142
    Metabolic Toxins 142
Metabolism 12, 27, 33, 61, 71, 137, 139, 142
Mindfulness 36, 37, 47, 48, 133, 142, 143
Mindset 26, 36, 46, 47, 49, 63, 143
Minerals 35, 37, 73, 78, 122, 129, 143

N

Negative Feedback 20, 143
Neurons 46, 140, 143
Neurotransmitters 49, 138, 143
Nourishment 32, 35, 37, 53, 78, 143
Nutrient 34, 37, 42, 66, 67, 79, 80, 81, 84, 90, 92, 93, 137, 143, 144
    Nutrient-Depleting Foods 34, 93
    Nutrient-Rich 90, 92, 137

O

Omega-3 37, 82, 89, 107, 143
    DHA 82, 143
    EPA 82, 143
    Omega-3 Fats 82, 143
Organic 35, 66, 77, 86, 92, 94, 102, 108, 109, 110, 111, 112, 113, 114, 118, 127, 129, 142, 143
Oxidative Stress (OS) 29, 143
Oxytocin 49, 144

P

Phthalates 35, 71, 144
Phytonutrients 35, 144
Pituitary 12, 19, 20, 137, 141, 144
    Pituitary Gland 20, 137, 141, 144
Preservatives 34, 67, 93, 144
Processed 34, 37, 66, 69, 140, 144
    Processed Foods 34, 37, 66, 140, 144
Protein 35, 37, 61, 67, 78, 82, 85, 86, 88, 90, 91, 105, 140, 144

R

Refined 34, 66, 67, 69, 86, 88, 90, 93, 137, 144
    Refined Foods 34, 67, 93, 137, 144
Rumination 22, 36, 46, 144

S

Self-Love 37, 41, 42, 43, 44, 64, 77, 84, 96, 99, 131
Sleep 18, 21, 25, 27, 32, 33, 39, 42, 47, 53, 54, 57, 58, 59, 61, 63, 86, 90, 122, 134, 139
Stress 11, 12, 13, 15, 16, 17, 18, 19, 20, 21, 22, 23, 24, 25, 26, 27, 28, 29, 30, 31, 32, 33, 36, 37, 39, 41, 42, 46, 49, 53, 54, 65, 72, 80, 131, 135, 138, 139, 140, 141, 143, 144
    Perceived Stress 25, 26, 46
    Stressor 20, 26, 29, 33, 36, 65, 138, 144
    Stress Signals 25, 144
Sugar 20, 25, 27, 34, 37, 61, 67, 68, 69, 70, 86, 88, 92, 93, 94, 105, 134, 139, 140, 141

Sucrose 68, 70, 145
Sugar Imbalances 25, 27
Supplement 72, 79, 80, 81, 82

T

Toxic 17, 18, 33, 34, 35, 36, 38, 65, 66, 71, 72, 73, 74, 77, 84, 133, 144
Toxic Foods 34, 66
Toxicity 33, 34, 35, 36, 65, 71, 73, 140
Toxic Load 71, 74, 77, 84, 133
Toxins 34, 35, 71, 73, 74, 142, 145
Transition Foods 34, 145
Tryptophan 33, 62, 90, 145

V

Visceral Adiposity 28, 145
Vitality 16, 25, 42, 53, 57, 75, 96, 98, 99, 145

Z

Zeitgebers 26, 27, 145

www.ingramcontent.com/pod-product-compliance
Lightning Source LLC
Chambersburg PA
CBHW071348080526
44587CB00017B/3011